THE GENTLEMAN'S GUIDE TO LIFE

WHAT EVERY GUY SHOULD KNOW ABOUT
LIVING LARGE, LOVING WELL,
FEELING STRONG, AND LOOKING GOOD

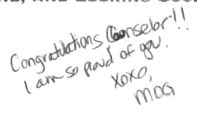

Congratulations Counselor!!
I am so proud of you.
XOXO,
MOG

STEVE FRIEDMAN
ILLUSTRATIONS BY MICHAEL CRAWFORD

 THREE RIVERS PRESS · NEW YORK

Published by Three Rivers Press, New York, New York.
Member of the Crown Publishing Group.

Originally published in hardcover by Clarkson N. Potter, Inc., in 1997.
First paperback edition published in 1999.

Random House, Inc. New York, Toronto, London, Sydney, Auckland
www.randomhouse.com

THREE RIVERS PRESS is a registered trademark and the Three Rivers Press
colophon is a trademark of Random House, Inc.

Printed in the United States of America

Design by Maggie Hinders

Library of Congress Cataloging-in-Publication Data
Friedman, Steve.
The gentleman's guide to life: what every guy should know about
living large, loving well, feeling strong, and looking good / Steve
Friedman; illustrations by Michael Crawford. Includes index.
1. Men—Conduct of life. 2. Self-realization. 3. Etiquette for men.
4. Success. I. Title
BJ1671 .F75 1999
646.7'0081—ddc21   98-37679
ISBN 0-609-80202-X

10 9 8 7 6 5 4 3

CONTENTS

LIVING LARGE 13

Moving up without selling out, helping your friends, crushing your enemies, impressing strangers, and staying true to yourself.

LOOKING GOOD 55

You might be nothing but a naked ape, but don't you want to be a well-dressed, clean, groomed, stylish naked ape?

FEELING STRONG 91

Your body is a temple. Don't be a heathen.

LOVING WELL 127

Is she the woman of your dreams, or are you having a nightmare? And how can you find true love without losing lust?

ACKNOWLEDGMENTS

I'd like to thank my agent, Chris Calhoun, and my editor, Annetta Hanna, for making *The Gentleman's Guide to Life* possible. I'd also like to thank, for their expert and wide-ranging research assistance, Joseph Amodio and Jeannette Batz Cooperman.

For their tolerance and understanding while the book was written, GQ's editor-in-chief, Art Cooper, managing editor, Marty Beiser, and executive editor, David Granger.

For her design talents and great sense of style, Robbin Gourley. For his wise and weird drawings, Michael Crawford. For his generosity and darkroom wizardry, Nick Kelsh. For her design, Maggie Hinders.

For advice, suggestions, expertise, and help on matters legal, romantic, culinary and everything else: Mark Adams, Joe Bargmann, Frank Bouting, Eileen Bugnitz, Richard Ben Cramer, Mary Duffy, Raymond Farruggia, Ann Friedman, Don Friedman, Maura Fritz, Ken Fuson, Nichelle Gainer, Mary Ann Gwinn, Lisa Henricksson, Dr. Helen Henry, Tom Junod, Katherine Kane, Terrell Lamb, David Lance, Jeff Leen, John Limotte, Connie McCabe, Terry McDevitt, Adrienne Miller, Jim Moore, Robert Moritz, Robbie Myers, Scott Omelianuk, Curt Pesmen, Alan Richman, Ruth Rosenbaum, Alex Ryshawy, Connie Saint, Al "Freddo" Scotti, Jennifer Scruby, Suzanne Steele, Sarah Tucker, Carolyn White, Catherine Wible, and Mary Wible.

And for her patience, good humor, support, affection, and enduring friendship, Leslie Yazel.

To sensible men, every day is a day of reckoning.

—JOHN W. GARDNER

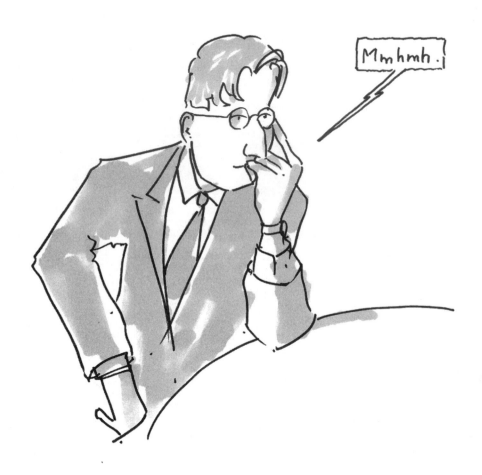

INTRODUCTION

Let's say you're the kind of guy who aspires to a certain kind of life—one abounding with material success, satisfying work, exciting and enriching romance, empathy for others, connection to God. Let's say you admire Great Men and strive to do Great Things. Let's say your role models are Genghis Khan and Attila the Hun.

Or maybe you're the sensitive type, in touch with your spiritual side, more finely attuned to your nurturing instincts. In that case, the would-be world emperor for you is Napoleon "Who You Callin' Shorty, Bonehead?" Bonaparte. Or King David, who in addition to coldcocking Goliath and keeping peace in the Middle East, also had the street smarts to order the husband of his girlfriend (Shalom!) into battle.

Myself, I've always been partial to Gandhi, Billy Jack, St. Francis of Assisi, Bronco Nagurski, and the Angel of Death. Also Babe the Blue Ox and Jesus, too, but wouldn't it have been cooler (and more manly) if he had used his superhuman powers to turn his enemies into loaves of bread or something?

The problem is, emulating even the greatest historical figure carries certain inherent liabilities. I mean, you can go with the Fu Manchu on your face and utter ruthlessness in your day-to-day behavior, but without some Mongol hordes to watch your back, you're nothing but a funny-looking sleazebag. The battlefield tactics of the stubby-legged French warrior still fascinate you? Try shouting "L'audace, toujours l'audace" the next time your boss tells you that your latest proposal would expose the company to lawsuits, bankruptcy, *and* public humiliation. Not exactly a *très bonne idée*, half-pint.

No, history is fine, but if you're like most guys, you run into contemporary problems that would confound Confucius, perplex Plato; riddles and mysteries that would baffle even Bill Moyers.

Matters of the heart? You love your girlfriend, but the idea of sex with her younger sister is not exactly, um, *foreign* to you. What about fashion? Single-breasted versus double-breasted? Spread collar versus button-down? Cuffs? Sure, the founders of the Judeo-Christian, Muslim, Buddhist, and Hindu traditions who have been guiding and strengthening the human race for thousands upon thousands of years might have been perfectly content in nothing but robes and sandals and beards, but use your head—these guys were *market leaders!* Think they didn't pay attention to styles? You *know* if Moses were around today, he'd be wearing Polo. (Not to mention chowing down on a nice piece of brisket. Forty *years* of manna? Gimme a break. I don't care if it *did* come from heaven.)

These days, the ability to tote stone tablets is nice, but not enough. These days, the measure of a man means much more than "40 regular." These days, everyone from atheists to Zen Buddhists needs to know about clothes, about grooming, about business, about romance, not to mention meaning and a profound sense of peace and happiness and what's the best way to squash that human cockroach in the cubicle next to you.

With apologies to Thomas Paine, *these* are the times that try men's souls. Lucky for you, the answers are at hand. Sometimes the solution is simple (regarding your honey's sister, look, but never, ever, *ever*, touch). Other times, you need more information. (Flat-front khakis are fine for lean and hungry types like Cassius, but if you're built like the Buddha [the fat one], think pleats.)

Why trust me to deliver the goods?

Because in addition to editing, assigning, writing, and generally serving as majordomo of GQ's health and fitness section for the past four years, a time in which I have become an expert on subjects ranging from aerobics to yoga, breathing to spiritual fitness, cunnilingus (I edit the sex column) to "weightless" workouts, I also possess the rich and fecund life experience of Everyguy. In spades.

I have fired and been fired, wooed and been wooed, dumped and been dumped. I also once dated a famous advice columnist's granddaughter and consequently absorbed a lot of useful information until the unfortunate evening I referred to Grandma as "old moneybags."

My maternal great-great-grandfather was a rabbi, his son a teacher, his son a lawyer, and his daughter ("Mom" to me) a psychotherapist, so I can tell a guy when he's spiritually adrift, legally at risk, *and* ambivalent about marriage (or at least pursuing his girlfriend's little sister for reasons that have more to do with unconscious desires than the pert way she flips her hair). On Dad's side, there's a tailor, a pharmacist, and a financial planner (aka "Pop"), so clothes, drugs, and money aren't a problem either.

Read this book and you'll learn how to leave them laughing and make 'em cry. You'll gain a better understanding of the relationship between alcohol and health as well as the one between honesty and career advancement (similar ratios, by the way, in which a little can go a long way). You'll discover the secrets on how to make a move, take a chance, proclaim your love, meet your girlfriend's folks, duck phone calls, advance your career, talk about art, make an excuse, apologize, and weasel out of an obligation (hint: do them one at a time).

Want to know if you're getting enough sleep (and how to get more)? Interested in learning how to find a shrink or why your girlfriend is *sure* you need a shrink? Want to buy a woman flowers, avoid gaffes in the sack, propose, get divorced, order wine, get a raise, lose weight, gain muscle, feel better?

Of course you do. And I'll tell you.

This is a book for a man who wants to live large, look good, feel strong, and love well. Read it, use it, learn by it. Above all, forget your girlfriend's little sister.

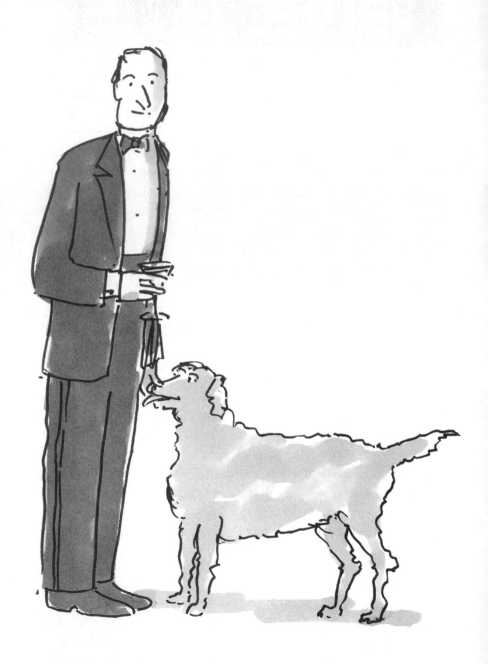

LIVING LARGE

Money can't buy happiness, but you sure as hell better have enough to pay the rent for a really nice one-bedroom apartment. And while peace and fulfillment come from within, a corner office with a nice view and company tickets to the local ball games don't hurt either.

Corkscrew, a ticket broker, some choice CDs, books that address the most critical aspects of manliness, the name and phone number of a good therapist.

How much is enough? How much should I tip? If ignorance is bliss, how come I'm not kicking up my heels? What books should every guy read? How do I behave at someone else's dinner party? What's the best way to get ahead in business? How can I goof off at work without fear? Is revenge really a dish best served cold? What's the secret to success in cyberspace? Do I need a shrink, or are my plans for world domination reasonable? And finally, if I'm wealthy, successful, and wise, how come I don't feel better?

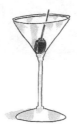

The key to living large

is not fearlessness. It is not raw knowledge, it is not even *savoir faire* or *joie de vivre* or a certain, oh, *je ne sais quoi* (though knowing how to drop French phrases like these from time to time will help on dates with women who wear black, sneer a lot, and smoke).

To live large, you must connect with others while remaining true to yourself. You should possess a finely calibrated sense of justice (an eye for an eye, according to the Old Testament) while feeling secure enough to turn the other cheek, the suggestion of another fairly well known religious leader. If you live large, you know that knowledge is power, but you're acutely aware that "in much wisdom is much grief; and he that increaseth knowledge increaseth sorrow." (In fact, if you are living large but earning low, you quote this bit of biblical wisdom after every one of those vexing moments when your boss/wife/girlfriend/mother/grocery store clerk/other fixes you with a grim stare and asks, "Don't you know *anything?*")

To live large is to move through life with a sense of purpose, but to be more than willing to accommodate despair. It is helping friends and crushing the particularly fulsome enemy. It is firing and being fired, trusting strangers but knowing when to sense danger. It is ordering wine, talking about art, E-mailing with grace, listening with good humor.

Living large is adopting a personal code and sticking to it. The code should be a little more multidimensional than "A man's gotta do what a man's gotta do" (doesn't that one smack of sawdust-covered floors and Confederate flags?), but perhaps not as, well, squirrelly as "We are all God's creatures" (so what? I eat God's creatures. I compete with God's creatures. I mock God's creatures).

No, the best motto for today's gentleman is not "Live and let live." (Too vague, and besides, are you really gonna show mercy to the guy who's trying to move in on your sweetheart?) It's not "Never play cards with a man named Doc, never eat at a place called Mom's, and never sleep with someone more screwed up than you" (not necessarily *bad* guidelines, just not inclusive enough).

Man's most credible credo for the coming millennium is, I submit, something along the lines of "To thine own self be true," as long as thine own self isn't a shifty bum who sleeps too late, drinks too much, and can't hold a job.

Wisdom can also be found in the wise and remarkably rich musings of those inexplicably underrated musician philosophers, the Fifth Dimension, who sang, "Do what you wanna do. Be what you wanna be. With whoever, you really wanna be with." The downside there is potential legal problems.

No, the bottom line for living large was revealed to me by a former boss, a well-respected and not so incidentally somewhat feared man. "To get ahead in this life," he told me one day, "there are only three qualities you need to possess. Everything else is mere sideshow. The first quality is decency. The second is honesty. And the third is integrity.

"And once you learn how to fake those, you're in business."

AT THE OFFICE

It pays the bills. It gives the headaches.
It offers the promotions.

Office politics

Work hard. Stay late. Give credit where credit is due. Make your company a better, more valuable place, and you will be rewarded. Eventually.

Or don't work so hard. Instead, hang out at the fax machine, looking for sensitive documents whose ideas you can claim as your own. Buy drinks for your colleagues and pry their computer passwords from them. Then hack into the office computer system and mete out justice in a way that might seem capricious and cruel to others, but makes perfect sense to you. Spend a lot of time with the big man. Call him "big man." You will be rewarded, or fired, and it will be fairly quick. You will also be despised.

Goofing off

This is best practiced when you work for someone. If you're your own boss, goofing off isn't as daring, as dangerous, or as much fun, unless you have some deep-seated and profound identity issues. The problem with goofing off is, you'll probably get caught. Here's how to minimize the downside.

Always look purposeful. You check groceries for a living and you're headed to the loading dock to sneak a beer with the manager's teenaged daughter? Carry a clipboard. When someone asks, you're on your way to "take inventory."

Ogling the "I'm not worthy of Isabelle Huppert" page on the Celebrity Babes of the Internet? Ogle with a steely gaze, and a slight frown. You are serious, you are sober, you care about this company, and most important of all, you have made sure to position your desk in such a way that no one from the hallway can see your computer screen.

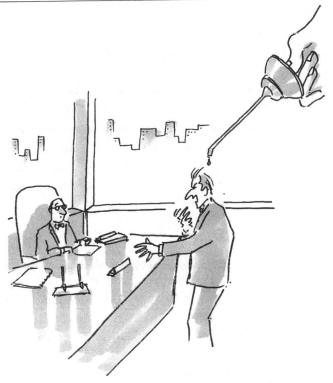

The squeaky wheel gets the oil. Or he gets greased.

The boss calls you into his office one day and wants to know about the $1,400 in long-distance bills you have racked up in the past three weeks to a certain telephone number in Lawrence, Kansas? Do you tell him that you have been pitching woo to a Jayhawk cheerleader you met at Club Med last summer, and with whom you feel a strong bond? No.

Instead, stress her university affiliation and her area of study (no need to mention she's a sophomore) and how "interfacing" (use this word only in emergencies) with her can help your company. "I've been dialoguing with a Kansas University economist [he doesn't need to know it's Economics 101] about cost-saving and productivity-enhancing measures in the marketplace" might save you.

Finally, if you're busted, stand tall and say these words, also basso profundo: "It was a judgment call, boss."

> *Does saying to some guy you hardly know,*
> *"Great job on that report, Fred, and by the*
> *way, you gotta tell me how you stay in the*
> *shape you're in, you're a* rock, *and that's an*
> *incredible suit, you look like* you *should be*
> *running this place," really make him like you*
> *and trust you more?*

Yes.

The care and feeding of the boss

You've been told that the squeaky wheel gets the oil. But you've also heard to keep your eyes open and your mouth shut. So what happens when you're ready to make a brilliant move that will help the company and delight your boss, but you're worried about the cost involved in said move, and the slight chance it won't work. Do you follow the dictum "It's easier to get forgiveness than permission" and forge bravely ahead? Or do you heed the slightly more forbidding "Never surprise your superior" and cower safely, but miserably, in your cubicle?

What's that? You say you're a man, dammit, not some grub-eating rodent? You're not going to spend your professional life living in fear? You will forge ahead, and you *will succeed?* Bravo, I say.

Until your plan fails.

Now, do you shift blame to your hapless and trusting, but not all that smart, cubicle partner who is blissfully unaware that the paper trail you have left points the finger at him? You say you're too decent for that, and besides, you didn't *remember* to leave a paper trail dooming your fellow rodent?

Then do you tell the big man you've made a mistake and are prepared to suffer the consequences? Do you call him "big man" while your chin quivers and your voice, just yesterday so powerful and un-rodent-like, quakes? Do you say, "It was a judg-ment call, boss," in a basso profundo that suggests that any secure captain of industry who doesn't appreciate underlings willing to make judgment calls is the kind of man who probably uses lip gloss?

Basically, it depends. Do you work for someone who encourages risk-taking and tolerates the occasional glorious failure? Or is he someone who likes his employees to play it safe? Tailor your actions accordingly.

Does he prefer written communication? Give him memos out-lining your plans. Is he a person who responds best to face-to-face discussion? Talk to him about what you're planning. Is he cranky in the morning, but full of enthusiasm after lunch? Now you know when to bring up that risky but promising plan of action.

In general, bring him completed projects and proposals, not half-assed beginnings, and when a problem arises, don't just tell him about it, suggest some solutions, as well. And never, ever go over his head.

Does he only reward employees who allow him to verbally horsewhip them? Does he call you Ted even though your name is John? It's time to look for a new job.

Things to avoid saying to your
assistant if you're ever lucky enough
to have an assistant
"You call this swill *'coffee'*?"

Making more money

Start with a good salary.

The way to do this is to find out the salary range of what other people in your position are making. Read Department of Labor quarterly reports; call headhunters. Ask trade and professional associations; use the Internet to poll perfect strangers.

Next, ask for the highest end of the salary range you discover. Remember, they want you. Also remember not to tell your prospective employers what you're making now. When they ask, tell them, "I don't think my salary at present is nearly as relevant as the work you want me to do in the position we're discussing, and I think the salary for that position should reflect that work."

If they press, inflate your current salary as much as you can without giggling nervously.

After you've been in a job for awhile, negotiate for a raise, and be creative.

The boss absolutely won't budge on that 2 percent increase? Then push somewhere else. How 'bout an extra week of vacation, some unpaid leave, increased educational and training opportunities? And as long as you're thinking, what about making your higher salary contingent on the company's increased profits? You're not asking for free money, you're merely asking for just compensation. So if your sales increase by 40 percent, you'd like $5,000 extra.

Do a great job.

A sad note: It's amazing how many people think they're entitled to more than a cost-of-living raise merely because they show up. Most companies do not function like the post office. A merit raise is supposed to reward merit. So be meritorious.

Get an offer from another company.

How to make friends at your new job

Say, "Hi, my name is Steve, what's yours?"

Say, "Great-looking tie there, pal."

Do not say, "Who do I have to blow around here to get something done?"

Getting fired

It doesn't matter if you deserved it. It doesn't matter that you need this job. It doesn't matter that you've given the damn company your heart and your soul. No, what matters is this: You need to make them as ashamed and afraid as possible, and you need to do it the moment the ax falls.

(Resist the impulse to feel afraid or ashamed yourself. You'll have plenty of time for that later.)

Before getting into shame- and fear-inducing behavior, and how you can get your executioners to jack up the amount of walking money they're throwing at you, let's examine the exact reasons you're being, uh, downsized.

Were you sleeping with the boss's daughter? Did you steal money from the company? Have you been taking four-hour lunches, arriving late, leaving early, and spending a bit too much time with Celebrity Babes of the Internet? If you answered yes to any of these questions, pat yourself on the back for getting away with it for so long. Now, take what they're offering and start asking yourself if maybe you shouldn't look for a line of work more suited to your unique temperament and talents.

If, on the other hand, you are losing your position because the company has had to shrink its workforce, or because your department head has been fired and the new guy is bringing in a new team, or for other reasons that have nothing to do with your performance, then chances are someone at the top might feel bad about what's being done to you. That's good. You want them to feel *real* bad. And you want that bad feeling to translate into the largest possible severance pay possible.

Having been fired twice myself (hint: if you're an editor, I'd advise against telling your owner, "I'm running this magazine according to my tastes, and if you don't like the direction, you should find another editor"), I know how painful the process can be. Make your boss feel your pain.

So tell the human resources hit man that you appreciate the company's position, but you really feel that your five years of service merit more than two weeks' severance, and you would appreciate his discussing a possible upgrading of your severance package with the appropriate people.

As for fear, the only trump card you hold here is what you might tell people in the community about the company. Mention the "company's reputation in the community" and your friend at the local paper doing a story on how "corporate citizens treat their employees." Chances are, no one will believe you, but you might get lucky.

Ducking phone calls, making excuses, apologizing, weaseling out of an obligation

Don't.

Don't.

Do, and with feeling.

Don't.

Firing

First, try to avoid it. Truth be told, firing someone is often the easiest solution to an otherwise solvable problem. It can also be the laziest and least decent. Maybe your employee isn't doing a good job because he doesn't know how to do a good job (and what idiot hired him?). That means you have to be a manager. Tell him what he's doing well. Tell him what he's not doing well. Tell him how you expect him to change his behavior and job performance.

This is not easy. It's called managing people. It's what you're paid for.

If you've done all that and you've still got to get rid of the guy, then your conscience shouldn't bother you. But what if you need him to finish a project/report/big deal?

The cold-blooded and all-too-common corporate answer is to let the poor dolt keep working until you have hired his replacement, or until his project/report/deal is done, then ax him. This is effective, but in the same way Mussolini was effective in getting the trains to run on time. And look how Il Duce ended up.

I'd suggest a more charitable approach. I had to fire a department head once. He knew I was going to fire him, I knew it, and we both knew I needed him for a while. I gave him a generous two months' notice, but warned him that at the first sign of bitching and moaning he'd be gone.

This carrot-and-stick offer worked well. But if it doesn't, you should have a backup plan ready.

If it's a more cut-and-dried, thanks-and-get-outta-here deal, be as honest and as gentle as you know how.

Do it in person. Don't lie. Be generous. And if possible, do it in a neutral office. If you do it in his office, he'll feel more comfortable spewing obscenities at you. If you do it in your office, you can't get up and leave and say you have to be somewhere else.

Don't tell the person how hard this is for you. He's the one it's hard for. Also, avoid the impulse to assure him that this might be the best thing that ever happened to him. It might be. He doesn't need to hear it from you.

Knowing when to quit

If you're nauseated every morning at the thought of going to the office; if Sunday nights are horror shows; if you've taken three months of mental-health days in the past two years; if friends, family, and strangers ask you "What's wrong?" more often than "How's it going?"—start polishing your résumé

IN THE WORLD OF IDEAS

Speaking with confidence, feeling with passion, judging with discrimination. Pretending with conviction.

Talking with confidence about art

The most important thing to remember is that great art often evokes a violent and visceral reaction. Also, a lot of the time it's about sex. So if you can manage, when discussing an exhibit with a date, to work the phrases "violent and visceral reaction" as well as "it speaks to me" into the conversation, you're on your way. If you have absolutely no clue as to what you're looking at, or what violent and visceral reaction you're supposed to be experiencing, talk about the painting's "ineffable effect" on you. Look sad when you say this.

If you keep this charade up for a long time, of course, you will be found out. Besides, art is *good* for you. Don't you want those violent and visceral reactions? Well, then, you need a little background.

We'll start in the 1860s, because that decade marked the beginning of the impressionist movement, and, many say, the beginning of modern art. Anything earlier than that can be covered with a hushed comment about the painting's "primal beauty."

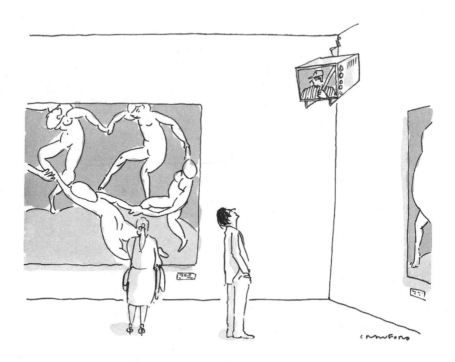

Looking at art.

Impressionism

The basics: The impressionists tried to capture a fleeting impression of nature, as if seen for the first time. They developed techniques based on the way the eye perceives light and movement. The paintings tend to blur up close; step back a few yards and the image crystallizes.

The big guys: Claude (the water lilies guy) Monet, Edgar (ballerina guy) Degas, Pierre-Auguste (like the water lilies guy without all the colors) Renoir, Édouard (the guy who liked tough, naked hookers) Manet.

Fun fact: An ophthalmologist wrote a few years ago that Claude Monet's paintings, which got blurrier and blurrier as he got older, showed not an increasingly fervid embrace of impressionism's tenets, but simply strong evidence of cataracts.

Postimpressionism

The basics: These guys painted as if the impressionists were wimps, because they thought they were. Starting in the mid-1880s, they went for more color, richness, and emotion.

The big guys: Vincent van Gogh, Paul Gauguin, Paul Cézanne, Paul Signac, Georges Seurat.

Fun facts: Van Gogh got really Postimpressionist with his ear only later in his career, after he moved into expressionist work. Paul Gauguin abandoned his family to capture, artistically speaking of course, all those hot island babes. And though Seurat is usually housed with the impressionists, his distinctive technique of pointillism was based on highly specific and precise color theory. If you can manage to say "distinctive technique of pointillism" or "highly specific and precise color theory" without cracking up, you can skip the rest of this section. You're already a master.

Symbolism

The basics: It's all about feelings.

The big guys: Odilon Redon, Edvard ("*Aieeeeeee!!!*") Munch, Henri Rousseau, Dante Gabriel (Mr. Pre-Raphaelite) Rossetti, Egon Schiele, Gustav (if there's gold in it, it's Gustav) Klimt.

Fun facts: That couple looks like they're arguing over what to eat? Hey, it's symbolism, it can mean whatever you think it means.

Fauvism

The basics: In French, the word means "wild beasts" and was used to describe a group of French artists who used violent, uncontrolled, brilliant color.

The big guys: Henri Matisse, André Derain.

Fun fact: "Wild beasts." 'Nuff said.

Surrealism

The basics: Taking its cues from Sigmund Freud's theories about the subconscious, surrealism worked within the world of dreams, fantasies, and images. The movement began officially in 1924, when the first surrealist manifesto declared the artist's duty to free man's unconscious personality from social conditioning and the rational ego's inhibitions.

Big, weird guys: Salvador Dalí, René ("Let's roll a reefer") Magritte; Joan Miró (a man, not a woman).

Fun facts: Salvador Dalí also designed ties, but their images were so sexual and violent few would agree to sell them. Later, he helped with Alfred Hitchcock's *Spellbound*, a psychoanalytically lush thriller with Ingrid Bergman looking hot while probing Gregory Peck's subconscious. And here's a bonus art joke to impress and amuse your Magritte-loving friends.

Q: How many surrealists does it take to screw in a lightbulb?
A: Fish.

Cubism

The basics: Its practitioners were determined to liberate form from its traditional representation. They emphasized the basic geometrical structure of the objects we perceive, beginning with still life and collage, and culminating in Marcel ("Daddy Dadaist") Duchamp's famous *Nude Descending a Staircase*, the scandal of the legendary Armory Show that brought Europe's new work to New York in 1913.

The big guys: Pablo (the guy was a complete hound with women but it doesn't matter; they love him anyway) Picasso, Georges Braque, Juan Gris, and Fernand Léger.

Fun fact: Even if you can recognize Picasso's work with ease, do not exclaim, when passing one of his paintings, "He's the Man! He's the Man."

Abstract Expressionism

The basics: The spontaneous, emotional, free-form paintings that made the art world notice America for the first time.

The big guys: Jackson Pollock, Jasper Johns, Marc (the blue donkeys and flying violin guy) Chagall, Edward Hopper, Piet ("Square Man") Mondrian, Mark Rothko, David Hockney, Francis Bacon, Anselm Kiefer, Wassily Kandinsky, Kasimir Malevich.

Fun fact: Edward Hopper influenced a generation of filmmakers. The house on the hill in *Psycho* was inspired by the Hopman.

A word of warning: "Once you learn terms, don't throw them around to impress people. Categorizing by school is very risky," says Teresia Bush, senior educator at the Hirshhorn Museum in Washington, D.C., which houses modern art for the Smithsonian.

Bush suggests reading a few classics, such as Janson's *History of Art* and Helen Gardner's *Art Through the Ages*. She also recommends that a guy "probe old bookstores and build up an art collection. Buy things you like, especially at the beginning. Adopt an art student and begin collecting (his or her) work you like."

Bush's advice is sound, of course, and her suggestions no doubt will lead to rich, hard-earned pleasures that can be gained only by the genuinely curious.

So remember, you can probe old bookstores, throw your money at dusty paintings, and "adopt" some art students. Or you can spend your weekends watching the classic sports channel and remember to say *ineffable* a lot.

Sounding smart about anything

Honesty is the best policy, naturally, and owning up to the gaps in your education is the morally upstanding thing to do. But neither will get you far in certain circumstances. That's when you need a mastery of some surefire buzzwords.

Say *derivative*. You can use this to comment on anything you have no clue about. It works especially well among New York City–based editors.

Say *jejune*. Be sure to sneer.

Say *gravitas*. This one is best used in the "It's got a certain..." and "It's lacking a certain ..." constructions.

Say *It's very smart*. This implies that you're secure enough to use small words, and open-minded enough to actually be enthusiastic about something. Best used in conversations with people from the Midwest, especially ones who have been hanging around New York City–based editors for any length of time.

Say *hopelessly nihilistic*. Translation: What a downer.

Say *He's quite the wunderkind*, but be sure to pronounce it *vunderkind*. Translation: He's young and rich and you hate him, but you're sophisticated about your hatred.

And when you want to dress up some run-of-the-mill chatter with an acquaintance, say *entre nous*. For example, "*Entre nous*, my girlfriend bores me, and when I look into your eyes, I feel a certain violent and visceral, but ineffable, something." It's better than "Just between youse and me."

The written word

Forget Conrad, Hawthorne, James, Allan Bloom, and John Updike. Of course you should read the masters and be conversant in themes of great literature. But this is the end of the twentieth century. And you're an end-of-the-twentieth-century kind of guy. Herewith, what you need to own and read about guy themes, like war, politics, meaning, drinking, drugs, crime, and growing up.

War

All Quiet on the Western Front by Erich Maria Remarque
  Dispatches by Michael Herr
  A Bright Shining Lie by Neil Sheehan
  Buffalo Soldiers by Robert O'Connor
  Catch-22 by Joseph Heller

War might be hell, but it's also great literature. Remarque recounts the horrors of World War I (from a German soldier's point of view). Herr serves up Vietnam in a druggy, rock-and-roll idiom that perfectly matches (and some say fictionalizes) the lives of the grunts he crawled with. Sheehan tells of the great intentions and tragic consequences of the same war through one soldier's career. O'Connor centers his tale of a peacetime American regiment around a likable heroin addict and pusher who falls in love with a one-armed teenager. Joseph Heller is said to have explained his work thusly: "It was written after the Korean War, set in WWII, about Vietnam."

O'Connor's is the funniest.

Politics

All the King's Men by Robert Penn Warren. Warren spins an American tragedy out of the life and times of demagogue Huey (Kingfish) Long.

What It Takes by Richard Ben Cramer. With the 1988 presidential campaign as his subject, Cramer takes the heretical position that the most successful American politicians are audacious, larger-than-life, and—most surprising of all—heroic.

Meaning

The Great Gatsby by F. Scott Fitzgerald. The nutshell: If you're an American, your dreams are unattainable, they can lead to the most destructive kinds of impulses, and they define you and make you great.

The Sun Also Rises by Ernest Hemingway. The first modern-guy novel, featuring rootless people trying to figure out how to live their lives and the one man who realizes the answer lies in creating a code and being true to himself.

The Snow Leopard by Peter Matthiessen. He's looking for the legendarily elusive snow leopard in the Himalayas. He never finds the cat, but he keeps looking, and looking and looking. Get it?

Love

Raymond Carver's "What We Talk About When We Talk About Love," "Cathedral," and "A Small Good Thing." Though it's fashionable to mock the minimalism and sense of loss that Carver wrote with and about, what the mockers miss is Carver's art and his profound sense of humanity. All these stories show the redemptive power of connection in the face of crushing loss.

Obsessive love

Endless Love by Scott Spencer. Guy loves girl, guy loses girl, guy's enduring love for girl leads to death, madness, destruction, and other bad things. Guy *still* loves girl.

Crime

The Killer Inside Me by Jim Thompson

Double Indemnity and *The Postman Always Rings Twice* by James M. Cain

Only Thompson could make a psychotic murderer/sheriff so likable. And only Cain could liken the feeling of looking into a murder accomplice's eyes to being in church.

Ryan's Rules (also released as *Swag*) by Elmore Leonard. Everyone loves Leonard now. Most haven't read this early work, which paired two friendly cons who set out to make a living by robbing grocery stores. They compiled their commandments for a successful career. One was "Be polite."

Drinking

A Fan's Notes by Frederick Exley

When the Sacred Gin Mill Closes by Lawrence Block

Exley's is a classic of denial. Block's is a detective novel about an alcoholic gumshoe named Matt Scudder. In later books, Scudder joins AA and goes to meetings while he's not nabbing bad guys. His life seemed richer, darker, and more interesting when he was spiraling downward.

Drugs

Bright Lights, Big City by Jay McInerney. Yeah, it's about a lot of other things, too.

Kings of Cocaine by Guy Gugliotta and Jeff Leen. The book that identified the Medellín cocaine cartel and told the story of the richest and most deadly group of criminals in history.

Newspapering

The Paperboy by Pete Dexter. Darkness reigns supreme, cynicism rules, and ugliness triumphs. And that's just in the newsroom.

Spies

Anything by John le Carré. You want moral ambiguity? He wrote the books.

Weird facts

Why Things Are by Joel Achenbach. Answers questions such as "Why do things get dark when they get wet?" and "What made the Beatles so great?"

Scientific explanation for why you behave like a sex-crazed pig sometimes

The Stone Age Present by William F. Allman. Bottom line: We're all animals.

Being a guy, albeit a gloomy, screwed-up guy

Anything by Robert Stone.

Just a few things you should know about music

That the Beastie Boys originally sang "We're going to fight for the right to party."

That women are fond of Leonard Cohen, the suicidal-sounding musician who did the sound track for *McCabe & Mrs. Miller*.

That some of the richest and most underrated music being produced today is Brazilian—you've got your native Brazilian influences, your African underpinnings, your Euroclassic harmony, and your American jazz roots. Plus it's easy to dance to.

Words to live by

I'm not going to tell you to buck up or to relax or that Rome wasn't built in a day or that he who hesitates is lost or some other superficially appealing but when-you-stop-to-think-about-'em kind of dumb philosophies to adopt.

No, what you need are words of wisdom that mean something in today's world. Here are a few.

For those times when you're working over the weekend while everyone else is on Rollerblades and having a grand old time, and you've already told yourself that "winners never quit, quitters never win" and that "if at first you don't succeed, try, try again," and you've even gone over the one about the ant and the grasshopper and silently chanted that "this, too, shall pass" and you still have a headache and want out, bad:

> *If at first you don't succeed, try again. Then quit. No use being a damn fool about it.*
>
> —W. C. FIELDS

For those times when your wife/girlfriend/pals/boss/child/inner child/mother-in-law, etc., says, "Jesus, are you ever going to get a promotion?" or otherwise remarks on how short a distance you have traveled on the corporate ladder, especially considering your age:

> *Neither necessity nor desire, but the love of power, is the demon of mankind. You may give men everything possible— health, food, shelter, enjoyment—but they are and remain unhappy and capricious, for the demon waits and waits, and must be satisfied.*
>
> —FRIEDRICH WILHELM NIETZSCHE

(It's best after you say this to sigh, smile wearily, and say, "That's from *The Dawn of Day*, though I don't imagine someone like you would be interested in that.")

Fine points of law to memorize
Ignorance of the law is no excuse. ("But, Your Honor, I didn't know she was only fifteen" will not help you. Neither will "I didn't see the speed limit sign.")

Oral contracts are binding in most states for $500 or less.

If you break it off, she often gets to keep the engagement ring.

If you're going to sign a prenuptial agreement, the further you do it from the wedding date, the less likely it is to be overruled. If your wife signs something the night before the big day, she can

always claim that that was under duress, as she was too "emotionally distressed" to think clearly. Some judges buy that.

People who give other people sexually transmitted diseases can
be successfully sued.

WHERE NOBODY KNOWS YOUR NAME

A loaf of bread, a jug of wine, a quiet table.

The secrets of ordering wine, distilled

You could spend the next ten years studying wine. You know people
who have spent the past ten years doing so. But living large is not
about sniffing a cork, sitting back, and proclaiming, "This is a well-
meaning and perky little grape, slightly promiscuous but in no ways
like the little slut we sampled the other night. Pour away, my friend."

You do, on the other hand, need to know certain things to order
with grace.

Know this:

White wines go with almost anything, except for fatty red
meats. And red wines, especially when they're young, served
slightly chilled, and don't have a high tannin content, get along
fine with most fish. Tannin is a chemical extract, produced by
grape skins. Heavily tannic wines overwhelm things like fish and
chicken, but they do a nice job of cutting through the fat with a
dish like a porterhouse.

"So don't drink tannic red wines with fish, or wimpy white
wines with steaks," says Alan Richman, GQ's food and wine writer,
and winner the past four years of the prestigious James Beard award
for magazine writing about food. "Almost everything else between
is not very embarrassing."

But shouldn't a gentleman be an expert on vintage years?
Shouldn't he be able to discern the subtle differences between the
northern Rhône and southern Rhône vineyards in 1983?
Shouldn't he be capable of discoursing at length on the subject of a

merlot's "nose" and the "bouquet" of a chardonnay, and how "the 1970 Montrachet from Domaine de la Romanee Conti is an absolute steal at four hundred dollars"? Let me ask another question: Would you want to sit next to a guy who could do all that, at dinner? No one else does, either.

When it comes to vintage years, get a chart from a wine magazine or a wine store. Memorize a few good years. Stick to them. For example, 1995 was a good year for most wines. So you're safe ordering anything from that period. As a bonus, you get to say, "That was a very good year," when you do so. If, as sometimes happens, a country's regions produce wines of markedly different quality in the same year, either drop that country or forget the year.

Drastic, yes. Useful, certainly.

That's for red wines. As for whites, don't order them if they're more than two years old (except for a few burgundies and German Rieslings and many of the best wines from the Alsace region of France, as if you even know where the Alsace region is). *Definitely* avoid old white wines from California.

Once you've decided on your 1995 burgundy, you need to order. One way to effortlessly blend your near-total ignorance with some always alluring savoir faire is to ask for the sommelier (that's "wine guy" to you and me).

Do not say, "What's your best stuff?"

Do say, "I know we'd like a pinot noir. Would you recommend a domestic or French? What's the best value?"

You are conveying some basic knowledge, a big dollop of humility, and a genuine concern that you not spend the month's rent on drinks. The sommelier will appreciate this and do you right.

When the wine is brought to your table, the waiter will pour a small amount in your glass and hand you the cork. First, though, he will show you the bottle. The most important thing to look for here is the level of the wine in the bottle.

If it's an inch or so below the cork, do not say, "Hey, what are we, getting rooked here?" Instead, mention, sotto voce, "The fill is a bit low. We'd prefer a high-fill bottle." You are not being greedy. Low fill is an almost sure sign that your wine has been poorly stored, or that the cork is defective. The wine might not be awful, but it sure won't impress anyone.

A bone-dry cork is another hint that the wine has been stored improperly. But it might mean nothing. So ignore it. (An exception would include the time you order something from the Alsace region and on the cork are written the words "Rocheport, Missouri.")

Next is the swirl, sniff, and sip routine. As you swirl, keep the glass in contact with the table. This way, you avoid "vertical vectors," which have to do with the ineffably fascinating physical properties of wine molecules. Also, you're less likely to spill it on yourself.

If you smell the wine and there's no odor, it could be it's too cold. It could also mean all the fruit flavor has been killed, which is one of the early signs of "corkiness," a condition imparted by a bacteria-infested cork. It could also mean there's just no smell. It's hard to say. So ignore this, too.

Now you let the wine sit gently on your palate. Many guys refer to this as "tasting the stuff." If it tastes like sherry, air has seeped in, oxidization has occurred, and you don't want it. (Sherry is deliberately oxidized wine.) If it tastes very, very musty, it is corked, and you're well within your rights to send it back. And if it smells and/or tastes like vinegar, you have discovered a bottle with "volatile acidity," which also provides solid grounds for refusing the bottle. The chances of encountering any of these problems is small, especially the last. But admit it, wouldn't it be cool to say, "I believe there's a volatile acid at work here, my good man. Perhaps another bottle would do better?"

You want to know more and refer to arcane facts? Read wine writers, check out *The Wine and Travels of Thomas Jefferson* by James M. Gabler, Bacchus Press (Gabler also authored a helpful tome, *How to Be a Wine Expert*), then quote from it selectively and spontaneously.

Familiarize yourself with a few terms such as *dry*, which means not very sweet, and *tart*, which means fairly acidic (but, rest assured, not in a volatile way).

Do not pronounce a certain wine "earnest" or "amusing."

Do not ever call a bottle "promiscuous" or "sluttish." You will fool no one.

Don't call the waiter "my friend."

Tipping

Shouldn't conscientious service be its own reward? Shouldn't waiters and valets and housecleaning help and parking guys and Chinese-restaurant deliverymen and everyone else in this great land of ours be paid a decent salary for a decent day's work, thus obviating the need to dig in your pockets each time someone does something nice for you?

Well, yeah, but shouldn't you be running your own company and married to Helen Hunt and spending your free time raising money for the homeless?

The moral is, the world is not a fair place. So once again, you need to learn a few basic rules.

When you go out to eat, 15 percent is the standard for efficient, friendly service. Twenty percent is reserved for really efficient, memorable service. Ten percent is what you leave when the waiter is actively rude, utterly indifferent, and/or spectacularly incompetent. You're well within your rights to leave less, but if you do so, it might cause a scene. Easier to avoid the place in the future. More emotionally cleansing to write the manager a letter.

Should you tip the contemptuous, bored, stoned, and hostile young person who charges you $1.30 for about two ounces of barely decent java at the neighborhood coffee bar? I have no position on this. You make the call.

When you're at a hotel, tip the bellman and the parking valet $5 or $10 each time they render service. If the concierge scores some great tickets for you, give him the same amount. Don't give anyone more than $20, unless you're a rock star or just dumb. And when you depart, leave an envelope at the front desk for the housekeeping staff. Two to three dollars a day is fair. Tip after the service is performed, not before. "A tip should be based on merit," says Frank Bowling, vice president and general manager of Los Angeles's Bel-Air Hotel, one of the world's preeminent hotels, home away from home for the likes of Cindy Crawford, John F. Kennedy Jr., and the Reagans. The exception, he says, is "in extremis, when you absolutely need to have good service."

If you find yourself in extremis, but with no cash, do what Bowling does. "Get to know the maître d'," he says. "Just go and introduce yourself. Say, 'Hello, my name is Frank Bowling and I'm here on business and I'll be using the restaurant quite a bit. Which table should I have?' And then you don't arrive with your guests and get put by the kitchen sink. It precludes any disappointment."

But remember, if you say, "Hello, my name is Frank Bowling," and it's not, you've defeated the purpose of this exercise.

Ordering a martini

Be direct, and be firm. Say "I'd like a Boodles martini, straight up, stirred, with onions, extra-dry," not, "A martini, please."

You want a classic martini? Order it dry, with gin and vermouth.

Classic martini ditty, from Dorothy Parker: "I like to have a martini, two at the very most. After three I'm under the table. After four, I'm under my host."

AMONGST LOVED ONES AND NOT SO LOVED ONES

No man is an island. And even if you're a hard-to-reach
mountain hideaway,
you will have visitors from time to time.

Why you should help your friends

Because they're your *friends*, you selfish bastard. Because virtually every codified system of belief worth believing in encourages its adherents to help others. Because the whole Ayn Rand thing is kind of creepy. Because you figured out the irony and pain in Simon and Garfunkel's "I Am a Rock" in junior high school. Because it feels good. Because Androcles helped the lion and the lion did Andy right when it really counted.

Because a part of you believes the whole karma deal. Because you *should*.

Whether you should crush your enemies

One school of thought holds that forgiveness is divine. Then again, the guy who preached that got crucified. So don't get mad. Get even. And take your time. Life is long.

Telling someone he drinks too much

Should you tell? On one hand, you care about your friend/colleague/family member. On the other hand, you don't want to seem pushy and you don't want to create a scene, and really, is it your business?

To answer the last question first, let me pose another. If your best friend was dying of a reversible, easily diagnosed, but terminal-if-untreated disease—say, some type of skin cancer—would you keep your mouth shut because you didn't want to intrude? So, yes, you should tell him.

Don't tell him when he's drinking. He'll ignore you, or he'll forget. Save the serious talk for a time when he's sober.

If you're pretty sure he'll deny he has a drinking problem (and denial is a hallmark of alcoholism), then it might help to include some other friends and family members. This is called intervention, it's rarely pleasant, and it might save the drinker's life. Call your local AA hot line or a nearby alcohol treatment center for advice on how to proceed.

If he tells you that his work is fine, tell him that a lot of alcoholics function professionally. Tell him you worry about his health and you're concerned that his drinking might mean he won't be alive much longer. Tell him you miss the friend he once was.

How to buy gifts for nephews, nieces, and other children

Don't try to get them the latest music or game, unless you watch hours of Saturday-morning cartoons, in which case you might consider seeking professional help.

Don't get them clothes. They'll hate them.

Don't get little boys toy guns. Mommy might not like it.

Don't get little girls Barbie dolls, especially the collector's edition models that bleat, "Math is hard." Mommy might really not like it.

Don't get books and educational CD-ROMs. Mommy and Daddy might like it. Little Buck (or Susie) won't.

Do give cash, especially for kids over four. Between two and four, they will be impressed by the concept. After that, they start counting.

Standbys that have stood the test of time include Lego, art kits, Play-Doh, and Adventure Toys made by Fisher-Price, sanitized versions of the incredibly violent figures that the little monsters really love. They'll like these and mom and dad will tolerate them.

IN YOUR HEAD

*If you can order wine, talk about art, read the masters, and
manage millions—and you're still unhappy—the answer might
lie elsewhere.*

How to know if you're drinking too much

Are there times you can't remember, because of alcohol? Do you
find it difficult to get through a day without drinking? Have friends
or family told you they're concerned about your drinking? Do you
miss work because of your drinking? Do *you* think you might be
drinking too much?

If you answered yes to any of these questions, you should lay off
the sauce for at least a while. You're not necessarily an alcoholic,
but you might be. One way to find out is to quit and see what happens. If you're miserable and can't function without lubrication,
consider Alcoholics Anonymous.

Therapy-schmerapy

Is your free-floating anxiety and murderous rage toward drivers
who cut you off an adaptive and reasonable response to life, or a
sign that you are reacting to deeper, darker problems? A trained
mental-health professional will be glad to answer that question for
you, for only $50 to $200 an hour.

Allow me to save you some money.

Find a therapist if you think the Unabomber went a little too
far, but he had the right idea. Get thee to a shrink if you're certain
that the woman who dumped you would definitely take you back if
only she could taste the new scrambled-egg dish you have named
in her honor, and that certainty has led you to mail her samples of
the dish on a weekly basis. Consider the couch if you've had diffi-
culty sleeping for more than a few weeks, if your anxiety is so
severe you have trouble breathing, if life seems unbearably sad, if

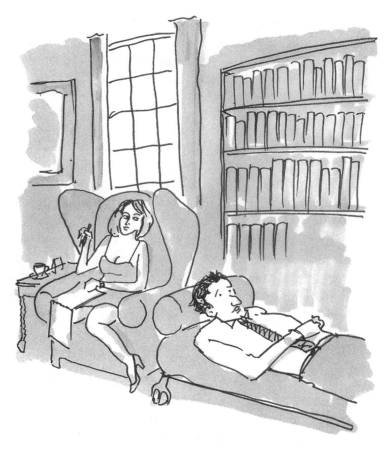

"Call me Mommy" means it's time to find another therapist.

you feel trapped, if the world seems like a mean and brutal place, especially during the weeks your home team is on a winning streak.

If your soul is thusly troubled, take heart: the stuff works. How? That depends on your therapist and his or her brand of therapy. One shrink might prescribe drugs to lighten your mood. Another might help you look more closely at the logic of your scrambled-eggs-dish-to-the-old-girlfriend scheme. Yet another might explore the roots of your anxiety and anger in your childhood.

In general, though, you'll do well to remember these guidelines:

"Do you hate your mother?" is an acceptable question from your shrink.

"You *should* hate your mother" is a little pushy.

"*I* hate your mother" is really too much.

"Call me Mommy" means it's time to find another therapist.

IN THE COMPANY OF STRANGERS

Sooner or later, you will find yourself in someone else's home. No matter what anyone tells you, do not "make yourself feel at home."

When you're a guest

Bring a gift and offer it when you arrive. This is not a bribe, but you hope it will serve as one. A bottle of wine is always safe, unless your hosts don't drink. If there are going to be other people there, bring food. Expensive coffee or a box of cookies from a chichi grocery works. If your hosts live in an out-of-the-way place like, say, Iowa, bring them something they don't usually get, like, say, Arthur Bryant's barbecue sauce from Kansas City or a half pound of lox from Barney Greengrass the Sturgeon King in New York City (they FedEx the fish in dry ice).

If you're in doubt, bring flowers. They might think you're clueless or resent having to stop what they're doing to arrange them—but they'll know you mean well.

Surviving someone else's dinner party

Eat. Unless you're going to have a terrifying, throat-closing, rash-swelling reaction to something, insert in mouth and swallow. Don't pick lima beans out of the three-bean salad. They're not gonna kill you.

Don't forget your table manners. With silverware, work from the outside in. Spoon soup away from you, and if you need to tilt the bowl to get the last drop, go ahead, but tilt the bowl away from you, too. If you need to get up during the meal, leave your fork and knife on the plate spread apart, tips angled toward the center, tines of the fork down. When you are finished, lay your knife across the upper rim of the plate, sharp side in, fork beside it on the inside, tines up or down. Do not belch loudly and proclaim, "Now, *that's* what I call strappin' on the feedbag."

Talk. It is your job to make conversation. You're not there to take up space and chow down. Ask questions, listen, and avoid the word *I* as much as possible. The other guests probably don't want to hear about your psychotic old girlfriend or the deal you're about to close. People like to talk about themselves. So let them. After you introduce yourself (loudly, as people tend to forget), try some of these tried-and-true conversational opening gambits:

"How do you know the host?"

"Did you read about those wolf attacks in India (or other news of the day, including but not limited to life on Mars)?"

"I saw the most amazing show at MoMA the other day. I just adore the fauvists."

"So, what do you do?"

But beware: In many parts of the world that question about occupation is the conversational equivalent of breaking wind. This is because, in many other countries, it is who you are, not what you do, that is important. This is a charming and humanistic way of looking at life. It also explains why we (us Americans, that is) live in the world's reigning superpower, and the charming and humanistic French guy next to you doesn't.

Do not bring up politics or religion or start a joke with "So, this rabbi and this priest went into a bar and . . ."

The one religion joke you might get away with is

Q: What did the Buddhist say to the hot dog vendor?

A: Make me one with everything.

(But don't say it if you're sitting next to Richard Gere.)

Do not look at your watch. Definitely do not shake your watch and look concerned.

Do not ask the woman seated next to you if she would like to
"blow this joint and go have some real fun."

Be nice. Do you have to bring a gift? Certainly not. But it will be
appreciated. Wine is always welcome (but you should not say,
when presenting it to the hostess, "Let's pop this bad boy and *par-
tay*").

Say thank you. A phone call is acceptable. A handwritten note
is nicer. It will ensure that you receive another invitation.

IN CYBERSPACE

It's a brave new world. Know the rules of the road.

No longer just the domain of skateboard-wielding hackers and
thick-lensed academics, cyberspace is where the modern man
checks sports scores from last night, reviews the Sherilyn Fenn
Worship Page, searches for the address and phone number of the
woman who dumped him fifteen years ago, and otherwise gets to
know his computer. Then there's E-mail, the communication
medium of choice for bankers and admen, friends and sweethearts,
and coming soon, your mother. (Now she'll have three ways to
remind you to set your clock back.)

E-mail

Cyber etiquette is crucial. Failure to comply marks you as a "new-
bie" (cybertalk for beginner) or, worse, an ill-mannered oaf. Only a
cad uses all caps. Only a fool writes in one mono-nightmare-lithic
paragraph.

So don't include the traditional letterhead lingo such as the
date, your address, sendee's address. The date and time will auto-
matically be included by the Internet postal elves.

And don't use all capital letters—it's tantamount to shouting
at someone. There are exceptions, of course. For example, "IF
THE YAMANACHI FIGURES AREN'T ON MY DESK BY

FIVE P.M., FIND ANOTHER SUCKER TO HIRE YOUR SORRY ASS" or "THE TV WAS A LOAN, NOT A GIFT. YOU CAN RUN, BUT YOU CAN'T HIDE."

Indiscriminate capitalization is less effective in this context: "HI, HOW'S THINGS IN DENVER?"

The biggest mistake you can make is to send an E-mail that might incriminate or embarrass you if your boss read it. It's lousy of him or her to read your mail; it's also legal.

The Net

Once you have a modem and browsing software, and you've logged about ten minutes of screwing around, you'll begin to see the possibilities. That's when you'll want the following addresses. Merely type them into the "location" space and you're off.

News

http://www.naa.org/hot/all.html

An alphabetical listing of every newspaper in the world that's on-line. Click on the newspaper you want, and go there.

Sports

http://ESPNET.SportsZone.com/

You know the score.

Relationships

http://www.swoon.co

The best on-line personals on the Web (they're free, too).

Sex

http://www.winbet.sci.fi/junkyard/sex.html

Everything and anything sex-related.

http://www.playboy.com

No brown-paper wrappers to worry about.
http://www.awpi.com/Combs/babes.html
An alphabetical listing of all celebrity-babe-related sites, from the official to the fetishistic.

Search engines

http://www.altavista.com
http://www.hotbot.com
http://www.yahoo.com

You want to find the phone number of your old college girl-friend? Curious about articles the past few years on quaaludes? Use any one of these.

Social commentary

http://www.suck.com

Written by a bunch of cynics who seem to think the Net was a better place when they were the only ones on it. Read their daily, often scathing attacks on technology companies or on-line media and impress your office's cyber-spewing, nose-ringed interns by knowing who's been "sucked" today.

Help

http://www.onlinesupport.com/

E-mail tales of your technical woes to these folks and they'll send you remedies and step-by-step guidance, usually within twenty-four hours. Sanity saving and easier than calling those pesky/tedious 1-800-help lines.

Tickets

http://www.ticketmaster.com

A national-events listing to help you plan your expenses-paid business trip to Chicago to coincide with Lou Reed's next Windy City performance.

AT HOME

No place like it.

B lack leather couches are nice, granted, as are fancy wineglasses, a laser-controlled CD player, and a fiftieth-floor private terrace and Jacuzzi. But all the comforts that money can buy don't add up to anything more than things money can buy. To be comfortable in your home, and make others comfortable there, too, you need to own things that speak to the heart and the soul, not just from the wallet.

The beat goes on—music you should own

Beatles or Stones? Mozart or Beethoven? Garth Brooks or Johnny Cash? Whether you interpret music as background noise, your life's sound track (you can't get out of bed without hearing the *Rocky* theme or "Born to be Wild"), or food for the soul, having a stack of vinyl or CDs that's well-rounded enough to merit being called "my collection"—as in "Would you like to come up and listen to my collection, my pumpkin flower?"—takes a little effort.

The Essential Johnny Cash (Columbia/Legacy 1992), aka *The Cash Box* (The ultimate coffee-table book of CDs. No wussy country here.)

Beck—*Odelay* (A modern classic of slacker, stoner hip-hop for the nineties. You're a loser, baby, if you don't have it.)

Duke Ellington: The Blanton-Webster Band (A three-CD set of jazz's greatest composer with his greatest band.)

Beastie Boys—*Paul's Boutique* (The first rap epic and the songs that saw these white, Jewish, fake-penis-wearing Boston beat-box babies reach music manhood.)

Elvis—*The Sun Sessions* (The sound of rock and roll being born. The King's early tunes such as "That's All Right, Mama," way before the jumpsuits and jelly doughnuts.)

Nirvana—*Nevermind* (Kurt Cobain: grunge messiah or analysis poster child?)

The Beatles—*A Hard Day's Night* (Guaranteed bad-mood buster. Proof this gang of four was more fun before they discovered drugs.)

The Complete Stax/Volt Singles, Volume 1 (The Bible of soul grooves from 1959 to 1968 from Motown's grittier Memphis cousin.)

Alex Chilton—*Like Flies on Sherbert* (This solo effort by ex–Box Tops, ex–Big Star pretty-boy singer was called flawed by those who swooned to the other bands' too-precious pop ballads. They were wrong.)

Elvis Costello—*Imperial Bedroom* (The perennial Brit before he started mistaking being clever for being good. The album he learned how to sing on.)

Ludwig Van Beethoven—Symphony No. 9 (Rousing. Powerful. Celebratory. All those adjectives you wish would occur to people when they thought of you. It sets Schiller's *Ode to Joy* to music and heralds the Romantic era. Plus, as a poignant historical note, the composer was deaf by the time he wrote this one.)

Gabriel Fauré—*Pavane; Pelléas et Mélisande; Masques et Bergamasques Suite; Fantaisie for Flute* (Gentle and dreamy without being cloying.)

Link Wray—*Rumble* (Brawny guitar. Instrumental rock. Quasi-rockabilly. Labels aside, it evokes the greaser era of ducktails, loud American motorcycles, leather jackets, and women in tight sweater sets.)

King of the Surf Guitar: The Best of Dick Dale and His Del-Tones (Surf guitar doesn't get better than this.)

Freedy Johnston—*Can You Fly* (Music you can feel coming from inside your chest.)

Hank Williams—*40 Greatest Hits* (As the song says, if you don't like Hank Williams …)

Anything by Billie Holiday and/or Ella Fitzgerald (Searing pain versus technically flawless scat singing. Both beautiful.)

Music to woo women

Frank Sinatra—*Songs for Swingin' Lovers* (A collection of Ol' Blue Eyes' snappy best from the days when women were called dames—if they were lucky.)

Van Morrison—*Moondance* (Mystical, sensual, watery.)

Carl Orff—*Carmina Burana* (Based on songs sung by dropouts from the early medieval clergy, this is divided into three long and weird poems about the coming of spring, drinking, and love. A spooky and arcane classic that works well with religiously inclined women.)

Marvin Gaye—*What's Going On* (It's political and sexy, but it's not a first-date album. Marvin moves slow.)

Al Green—*Greatest Hits* (Possibly the best soul singer ever before he discovered religion. His secular records are spiritual experiences themselves.)

Chris Isaak—*Forever Blue* (Derivative? Wimpy? Strictly a genre exercise? Yes, yes, yes. But an instant mood setter equivalent in date terms to a light-switch dimmer.)

Aaron Neville—*Warm Your Heart* (Sings like a girl but one with arms as big as your thighs, who soothes, soothes, soothes.)

Miles Davis—*Kind of Blue* (The pinnacle of small-group jazz improvisation and accessible to people who don't know jazz.)

John Coltrane and Johnny Hartman—*John Coltrane and Johnny Hartman* (Coltrane and the largely forgotten Hartman pair up for voice- and sax-led romantic ballads.)

Anything by Barry White or Teddy Pendergrass (Home. Run.)

Making a martini

The ideal glass is seven and a half ounces and cold. Placing it in crushed ice is okay. Chilling it in the freezer first is much better. Next, put ice into a larger mixing glass, shaker, or martini pitcher.

Depending on how dry you want the drink to be, make the gin/vermouth ratio anywhere from two-to-one to eight-to-one. Shake or stir according to your, or your guest's, taste.

When garnishing with a lemon, squeeze the lemon peel over the glass and allow a few drops of oil to land in the drink, then rub the peel around the rim. For olives, choose small, firm, pitted ones (no pimento stuffing). Olives go best with gin, lemons with vodka.

Throwing your own dinner party

Don't.

If you must, have it catered.

If you're doing it yourself, have a woman help you.

If, for some reason I can't possibly imagine, you insist on doing it yourself, follow these guidelines:

Make it brunch, not dinner. Expectations are lower, people are more relaxed, and you can end it more easily than dinner. At night, you can't claim you have to go someplace. Plus, you can always go with your scrambled eggs.

Keep it simple. "Thank God for those little jars of diced garlic," says Stephen Noonan, co-owner of the Manhattan-based Food Plus Catering, "and for cooked, peeled whole tomatoes, too. Why should anybody ever have to dunk a tomato in boiling water in this day and age?"

Warning: If you throw a dinner party, you might start talking like Noonan.

Pay attention to the little things. Cold salad plates. Hot dinner plates. Bread and butter plates. No television.

Surprise 'em. "Do the unexpected," Noonan says. "Garnishes, sprigs of mint on the sorbet, a stick of rosemary sitting up out of the salmon—nobody ever knows what it is, they're not used to seeing the whole branch, so it looks exotic. Parsley in the butter—and God, that couldn't be any simpler."

Be like a Boy Scout, which is to say, prepared. Do as much in advance as possible. Have the ice in the ice bucket, the cocktail

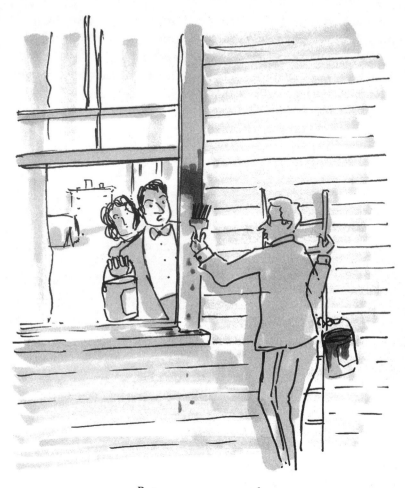

Put your guests to work.

glasses and wineglasses out, your first bottle of wine uncorked. Make your drink first, or you'll never get one. Wash up an hour or two before the guests come—you will always be able to boil water or slice bread, but you will not always be able to take a shower.

Remind yourself to keep it simple. "The soufflé is going to fall," says Noonan, "the hollandaise is going to lump. I usually find the after-dinner mints I bought days later—they got buried under things on the counter. Crab cakes are very simple, but everybody loves them, even people who don't like seafood. We serve them with wild rice and fresh, steamed vegetables."

Be deceptive. Candlelight makes it harder to see dirt and dust. When the brandy ice doesn't freeze, serve it as a little shake. If something didn't set, it's a soup. So don't tell anybody what you're serving until you bring it out.

Serve alcohol.

Get flowers.

Serve more alcohol (but have plenty of water and juice for nondrinkers).

Put your guests to work. "They'll be more comfortable if they're tending bar or putting on music for you," Noonan says. "And it breaks the ice when they don't know each other—they'll talk if they're both stuffing tomatoes."

Don't ask them to clean up. How would you like it?

Make everyone comfortable. If someone uses the wrong fork, you use the wrong fork, too. If someone takes the knife from the butter tray, let it go.

If you go buffet style, use the no-knife rule. Everything should be edible with only one utensil.

Work the numbers. Plan two parties in a row. Deep clean, hold a big formal party serving plenty of food, then have friends or family over the next night. The house will still be fairly clean, the flowers won't have wilted, and who needs to know you're serving leftovers?

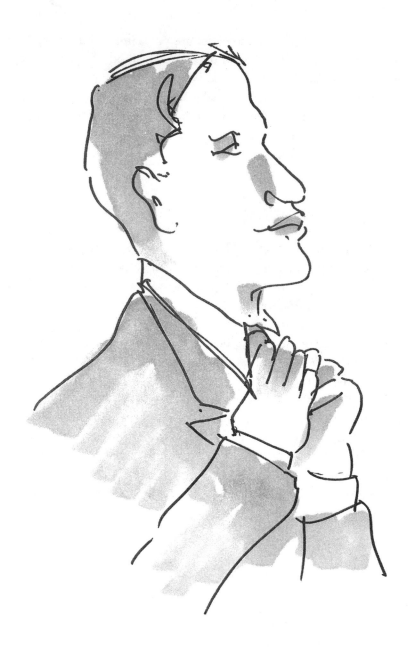

LOOKING GOOD

"Vanity of vanities, all is vanity," the good book tells us. And remember, less is more, except when it comes to spending money on a suit, in which case you always want to spend more than less. And, oh, yeah, floss everyday.

A navy suit, blue blazer, white straight-collar shirt, black and brown lace-up shoes, khakis, navy polo shirt, jeans, a tailor who knows your flaws and how to fit them, toothbrush, floss, nail clippers, leather dopp kit.

Can a man wear French cuffs with a sport jacket? What never goes out of style? Should shoes and belt match? Who can, and can't go double-breasted? Where's the best place for a monogram?

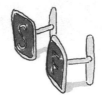

The apparel oft proclaims

the man," Shakespeare wrote.

"Looking goooooood, big fella," a colleague who wanted to borrow five bucks said.

"Wear that fucking shirt to the office one more day and you'll be taking a permanent vacation," a former boss informed me.

Each three of these extremely heartfelt sentiments reveals the powerful and subtle forces that shape the way men dress, shave, and comb their hair. It is those same forces and our fear of them that explain why so many fashion and grooming "experts" these days earn enough to sit at home in baggy shorts and T-shirts, sipping mango juice and chuckling away at their keyboards, telling the rest of us how to put on our pants and wash our faces.

Pick up a book or turn on the television and you, too, can learn how an almost indiscernible difference in the shade of your blue suit will help you escape from that dead-end job and land you in a corner office. Or for the price of a weekend on the beach, you, too, will become privy to precisely what cut of collar will grant you enormous power, which, if you're wearing the proper tie and applying the correct hair gel, you can wield with grace and kindness, only crushing underlings and competitors like worms when they deserve it, or if you just happen to be in a bad mood, or if the fellows are foolhardy enough to wear brown shoes with a black belt.

What these experts don't tell you is that many if not most corporations still operate under a simple and easy-to-understand code that you won't learn from any consultant. It is this: Ape your boss.

I don't mean "ape" in a pejorative or demeaning sense. Let me put it another way. At work, you are a valued contributor to a worthwhile enterprise. You are appreciated for your talent, your drive, your being. And, this is important, you are a trained monkey. The trained monkey who looks most like the Head Monkey will soon ascend the monkey ladder.

Some sociologists explain this phenomenon as the inevitable by-product of industrialized society, where large groups of men perform mechanized activities that lead to a common goal. (Thus the uniforms of armies, the Dallas Cowboys, and Republican speechwriters.)

Also weighing in on the whole do-clothes-make-the-man-or-just-make-the-man-funny-looking issue are the corporate anthropologists (read: guys who sip mango juice and wear baggy shorts) who dispute the entire notion of a sheeplike and crankily mewling workforce, pointing as evidence for their optimism to the ascendancy of Casual Friday and the large numbers of guys wearing denim shirts to their cubicles once a week.

Some of these corporate anthropologists theorize that the *fin de siècle* heralds a time of liberation and abandon, and that as the millennium approaches, American men are adding to their goals of pursuing life, liberty, and happiness the inalienable right to look cool and feel groovy.

They're wrong, naturally, but what do you expect from a guy whose job description is "study cubicle behavior, sip mango juice, come up with ideas"?

No, the "new relaxed but bold look sweeping the corridors of business," as fashion magazines have described it, has more to do with the aging of a population that was weaned on the idea that how it felt mattered. These baby boomers, dewy-eyed and potbellied now, have reached the point in their lives where they want meaning, fulfillment, and a lot of other things the Head Monkeys

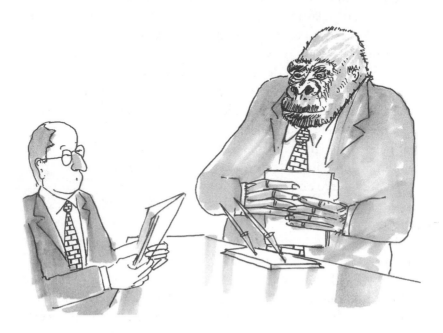

Ape your boss.

won't give them, including more scratch. (Head Monkeys don't get to where they are by acting like cuddly teddy bears.)

Instead, they figured a few years back that by allowing the sniveling pencil pushers to wear khakis and polo shirts one day a week, maybe it would keep them happy. It seems to be working.

So where does this leave you, an enlightened gentleman who wants to look good enough to be a Head Monkey one day but not so predatory that he'll startle the other beasts of burden? What does it all mean to a guy who can appreciate fashion and style but has a hard time embracing the wisdom of mango-juice drinkers? Does buying "loose fit" jeans make you a realist or a coward? Can a real man use moisturizer? And when the Bible says, "We are made a spectacle unto the world, and to angels, and to men," does it mean that even though a custom-made suit will set you back two months' salary, it's a good and religiously sound investment, and even if your wife doesn't approve, God does? And what's the deal on starch?

So many questions. Here come the answers.

SUITS

Gentlemen, prepare for battle.

No ad hominem attack conveys quite the same withering disdain as "You're just a suit." No epithet contains exactly the same degree of venom as "empty suit." No image evokes the absolute and lemminglike capitulation to the deadening yoke of conformity like "the man in the gray flannel suit."

So why wear them?

First off, because the Head Monkey wears them. Also, as Anne Hollander points out in *Sex and Suits: The Evolution of Modern Dress*, the suit "suggest[s] probity and restraint, prudence and detachment . . . [and] under these enlightened virtues also seethe its hunting, laboring, and revolutionary origins; and therefore the suit still remains sexually potent and more than a little menacing."

Um, yeah, and also because you want to get a raise.

What's the right suit for you, especially if the Head Monkey is a slob and you're dealing with clients all day, or if the Head Monkey is built like a real gorilla and your physique is more along the lines of Ichabod Crane? Or what if you don't have to worry about some antiquated corporate dress code (due to your enlightened Head Monkey or your trust fund or because you're a software designer), and/or style is something to which you aspire? What if you want something that actually feels good and looks smart?

In all those cases, your first step in buying a suit should be to visit one of the men's bulk discount stores sprouting like mushrooms along some of the toniest shopping avenues across the country. Price the low end of the store's suit selection. Next, multiply by four. A good suit is going to cost you at least this much.

Next, consider what the style writers, moody and stubbly cheeked male designers, and other people you wouldn't want to share a beer with have labeled the "sexy silhouette" in men's suits, a trend they swear will be around for many, many years to come, or at least for a few months. Question: Are you aiming for a "sexy silhouette" when you pull on your pants in the morning? I didn't think so.

Finally, look around you. Yes, you are an individual, and your unique and precious personality is screaming to get out. Well, let it get out, just not with a red-and-purple, four-buttoned number. (Heed the words of Flaubert, who said the wildest art came from the mildest artists. And remember that Wallace Stevens, one of this country's greatest poets, worked by day as an insurance executive. You can bet he wore suits.)

Color

Animals use colors to attract and to repel. You are an animal. The Bornean stinkbug is bright pink.

Savvy?

Bright colors, in addition to scaring people, make you look bigger and fatter, like a very large cousin of the Bornean stinkbug. In most circumstances, this is a look you want to avoid. So, especially if strangers feel compelled to exclaim, "Whoa there, big fella," when they see you approaching, and *definitely* if your nickname is Moose or Whaleboy or the Hog Who Walks Like a Man or some derivative thereof, stick with the charcoals.

Bright colors also draw attention. In most professional and social situations, you want to exude subtlety and a quiet mastery of the situation. Ninja assassins wore black. Bozo wore red and yellow. I think you can figure it out.

Blacks, gray (in many different shades), and navy have been around forever. There's a reason. They're classic. Khaki is fine for

summer and pinstripes and windowpane patterns tell the world
you're secure enough to be a little different. Other colors and patterns (including seersucker, which can be worn by some men and
shouldn't be by others) merely tell the world you *are* different. Be
careful.

Fabric

You don't know much, but you do know that polyester is for punks,
that shiny suits are best reserved for hit men, and that any label
that contains the word *Lycra* or *spandex* is a lining you don't want
near you.

Let's go back to the "you don't know much" part of that
thought. Advances in technology and the relentless march of fashion have changed things. Now many of the finest suits are made
with synthetics and blends. In fact, a wool suit with a small
amount of polyester will often keep its shape better and wrinkle
less over the course of a day than a suit of pure wool. The trick is to
make sure that the synthetic material is being added for endurance
and strength, and not as a cost-cutting device. The best way to do
that is to spend more.

It's also true that some very expensive suits are made of purely
synthetic materials, and that the shiny look is fashionable. I would
advise you to think of that look in the same way you think of sexy
silhouettes

You still can't go wrong with high-quality wool. The only cotton suit you should own is khaki, or seersucker (which used to be
made with cotton and silk, and is now cotton and polyester). Also,
remember that there is no such thing as a year-round suit. Ten
months, yes. But if you can wear it in the month of August, then in
January it rests.

Style

Most generally speaking, and that's going to be your language
when you're just learning, there are three basic styles of suits. The

classic American suit features a natural, untapered waistline, no darts, and what some would call a "relaxed guy" look and others would label "shapeless and sacklike." If you like your beer domestic, your clothes loose, and your movies action-adventure (and enough with the damned subtitles already), this is your model. Brooks Brothers will do you right.

A little more sophisticated? For world news, you only read the *Economist* and think baseball is "barbaric"? Then consider the classic European cut, which has squared shoulders, high armholes, a tapered waist, and tighter pants. (For this, you should possess, in addition to your ennui with boyish pursuits, a slim frame and flat gut.) To get a fix on this style, think Pierre Cardin in the seventies. Today, after Georgio Armani's loosening influence, it exists mainly as an archetype.

If, like most guys, you're somewhere in the middle, which is to say, you think of beer as "brewski," but you don't call it that in mixed company anymore, there is the updated American suit (made by designers of every nationality), with a slightly suppressed waist with lightly padded shoulders and added vertical seams to give shape. It's not as snug as the classic European, not as shapeless as the classic American. Calvin Klein, Joseph Abboud, and Ralph Lauren are three of the better-known names. Among these designers, Ralph Lauren's suits are the most traditional.

If you're tall and slender, you can get away with the classically European cut. If you're, uh, spectacularly not tall and slender, go with the classic American. Anything in between, you have more choices.

Add to these three standard models options such as two- versus three-button, single versus double-breasted, wool versus cotton, the question of jacket vents and pants pleats, and you can quickly become fair game for the salesman-on-commission who tells you that the linen number with the lime green stripes is "earnest and makes *such* a statement—now will this be cash or charge?"

Here's a quick primer:

VENTS Classic American suits usually have a single vent in the jacket. Classic British suits have double vents. Classic Italian suits have no vents. Vents these days serve little purpose, unless you have a big butt, in which case you need them.

BUTTONS A two-button suit can make you look slimmer because the drape of the lapels creates a V-shaped effect. Three-button suits can achieve the same effect, but only if the lapels "roll," or naturally meet, at the second button. The more fashionable three-button suits don't do that. "More fashionable" is another way of saying "there's a good chance that in a few years you'll want to throw away the photographs of you in it."

DOUBLE-BREASTED It's more formal, and it can add a barrel-chested look to even the slimmest-looking guy. Unchanging commandment: Keep it buttoned.

SUIT PANTS Regarding trousers, as the mango-juice crowd calls them (try saying *trousers* out loud to someone; I don't think you can), your best bet is double pleats and cuffs. Classic, comfortable, handsome. No sexy silhouettes.

The pleats should lie flat against your leg. If they're spreading (the pleats, not the legs), your hips are too wide and you need larger pants. Pleats make pants look dressier, they allow extra room (which you need if you sit down), and they hide things you shove into your front pockets.

Definitely go with cuffs. They add weight to the look. They're grown-up. The bottom of the cuffs should cover about two-thirds of the shoe length, and the cuff height should be anywhere from 1⅓ to 1⅝ inches. The taller you are, the deeper the cuff can be.

Fit

The collar of the suit should lie flat against the back of your neck and upper shoulders, allowing about a quarter inch of the shirt collar to show. Button the jacket (top button on a two-button, middle button on a three-button, all on a double-breasted) and sit down to see if the jacket pulls or appears to bulge. It shouldn't. Stand up again. Jacket sleeves should allow one-quarter inch to one-half inch of a dress-shirt cuff to show. An old rule of thumb (no pun intended) was to slightly curve your fingers, to make sure they just brushed the bottom of the suit jacket. Nowadays, just make sure the jacket covers your butt.

Still standing? Your pants should ride around your waist, not your hips. Look in a mirror. You should not be able to see your socks. Try walking. No one else should be able to see your socks. Worried about the slight horizontal crease near the bottom of the pants? Don't be. That's the "break." It's supposed to be there.

Now sit down. If you involuntarily say, "*Aaarrrrk,*" you might consider a larger waist size. Sometimes the jacket will fit almost perfectly and the pants not at all. That could have to do with the style of suit. The drop from chest to waist measurements in the American suit is seven inches, which means if you wear a 40 regular, you'll get pants with a 33-inch waist. In some European cuts, the drop is up to ten inches.

A good tailor can work wonders, especially with simple matters like shortening pants and letting out waists. But if a suit jacket puckers in the shoulders or drops too low or if it feels like a straitjacket—or if it's too short or too long—it doesn't fit. Translation: Take it off and try another size.

The details

Make sure the patterns match at the seams (especially lapels, shoulders, back center seam); buttons aren't plastic; buttonholes really work; and the collar lies flat. If there is thread wound round and round between fabric and button, the buttons were probably sewn on by hand. That's good.

Finally, check to make sure that the underside of the lapels has a felt backing, not a backing of matching fabric, and that all seams are secure and linings attached. Crumple the fabric to see if it bounces right back. When buying pants, make sure there's an extra button behind the fly area. This button takes the stress off the hook that keeps your pants up, and reduces pull on the fabric. Make sure the pattern matches in areas where two pieces of fabric are joined.

The case for custom-made

Say that you have a freakishly sunken chest or that one of your arms is longer than the other or that your skull is large, your shoulders broad, and your neck almost nonexistent. If you shop at a discount store, perhaps you've been made dimly aware of your plight. That's because on a few occasions you've heard salespeople shout, "Yo, here comes the skeleton" or "Who wants Lefty?" or "Heads up, human bullfrog in aisle seven."

The salespeople at most fine department stores and clothiers would never be so crass, of course. But even at those establishments, unless you're perfectly proportioned, your clothes will never fit exactly right, even with alterations.

Here's the real shocker: *No one* is perfectly proportioned. That's right, hyena boy, we're all freaks. You've just never realized it, because you've been buying off the rack your whole life.

All you need to do to discover how ill-fitting your suits are is to slip on a custom-made suit or shirt. Such an item, with its perfect fit, magic drape, exquisite cut, is enough to make you wish you had enough money to buy these duds the rest of your life. The problem is, you'd need a freakishly swollen checking account to do so.

A custom-made piece of clothing, in addition to fitting exactly right, is also made from the fabric you want, in the pattern you want, with the collars you want, and the pleats you . . . well, you get the idea.

If you're ordering a custom-made suit from a fine tailor, you will spend at least $2,000 and possibly much more. And if you have that kind of money to spend on suits, you don't need my advice.

If, on the other hand, you'd like the benefits of a custom-made suit—the style, the fit, the options, the sheer class of it all—without resigning yourself to lunches of peanut butter and crackers for the next five years, consider the made-to-measure suit.

Whereas a custom-made suit is made completely new—from whole cloth, as it were—when you get a made-to-measure suit, the design house takes a stock pattern, then adjusts it specifically and exactly to your specifications before creating your suit. Expect to pay about 20 percent more than an off-the-rack suit by the same designer would cost and expect to feel like a million bucks.

Cleaning

Don't even think about cleaning your suits yourself. Send them to a dry cleaner. You should be able to wear a suit at least twice before cleaning. Any more than ten or twelve times and you're pressing your luck. And speaking of pressing, unless you live in a hermetically sealed environment and/or don't sweat, you shouldn't get your suits pressed without getting them cleaned. Doing that will just seal in dirt. What you should do is invest in a brush, and use it on your clothes. Also, though dry cleaners will encourage you to clean your suits as often as possible, the fact is, doing so inevitably shortens the life of your clothes. So call the most expensive clothing store in your neighborhood and ask which cleaner it uses. Then send your clothes there.

Storage

Suits should be hung on wooden hangers. If you have air-conditioning and heat, leave your suits in unzipped plastic, to protect from dust and to allow air to circulate. If you live in a humid part of the country, consider no covering at all, because of the threat of mildew.

Some tailors offer their clients cloth suit bags, which offer the best of both worlds in protection and ventilation.

DRESS SHIRTS

*If you want to give someone the one off your back, it
probably doesn't fit right.*

It's next to your skin all day, unlike your suit jacket. It requires a
lot of attention, what with all the buttoning and rolling up of
sleeves and tugging at collars and spilling of coffee upon. And it's
the one article of clothing you actually wear where colors and
stripes and patterns aren't just tolerable, they're actually kind
of cool.

Color

White goes with anything. So does Milquetoast. Blue, long a standard among executives in Europe, has hit the mainstream in the
United States, and wearing a deep shade of it will mark you as daring but not subversive. Stripes, checks, and patterns? Life is risk.
Be a man. A careful man.

But regarding the white collars and cuffs on patterned shirts,
leave them for Head Monkeys like Ben Bradlee, who also happen
to be lions of industry.

Fabric

Buy pure cotton. It feels better than the cotton-poly blends, it
looks better, and the Head Monkey likes it better. Go for oxford if
you're on a limited budget and/or you insist on wearing T-shirts
underneath. It's the cheapest, most durable, and least translucent
of the cottons. The next step up is broadcloth, which is smoother
and silkier than oxford. At the top of the line are the most expensive, most delicate (so tightly woven they won't hold starch), and
most beautiful swiss cotton and sea island weaves. Oxford wrinkles
the least, swiss cotton and sea island the most. Stripes and patterns
"pop" the most in swiss cotton and sea island weaves, and least in
oxfords, where the cross-weave of color mutes the stripes.

Collars

You say your father wore button-down collars? You say that to your fundamentally decent self, the term *button-down* means "good," "caring," "a straight-ahead kind of fellow"?

These are noble sentiments, if you want to make a career out of being good and caring and straight-ahead. If you'd like to add "happenin'" and "possessed of some major disposable income" and "maybe he's an accountant, but he's a kick-ass, boss accountant" to the equation, say bye-bye to button-down. It's dowdy.

Take a long, hard look at yourself. No, not at the way your guts roil every night when you contemplate how you cheated on that book report fifteen years ago, man, your face! If your kisser is long and angular, you should opt for a full spread. If colleagues call you Al and they mean it as an affectionate diminutive of Alfred E. Neuman, go for at least a standard collar, which has points 2¾ to 3 inches long (measured from collar tip to neckband).

If you have a long neck, choose a raised collar; a short neck, a lowered collar. Tab collars are for the fastidious. Rounded collars for the very dressy Eton schoolboy look. Look for an unfused collar, in which the interfacing between the front and back linings is not glued to them. In collars with fused linings, in which the layers are glued together, the adhesive often crimps when the shirt is laundered, giving a "bubbly" appearance. "Ol' bubbly neck" is not the corporate moniker you're seeking.

Fit

Chances are, you have your shirt measurements down cold. Chances are, they're the wrong ones. The sleeves should end at the point where the wrist joins the thumb. The buttoned collar should not make you gasp or turn purple. The body of the shirt should not hang on you. Neither should it make you look like a cast member from *Saturday Night Fever*. And remember, a cotton shirt will shrink after its first cleaning. So give yourself an extra half inch in the neck and one-half to three-quarters of an inch extra length in the sleeve.

The details

You're going to need collar stays and you're going to lose collar stays. To replace them, go to almost any decent men's clothing store and they'll give you a bunch for free. If you want to splurge, get a leather carrier filled with brass stays.

If you're going to get a monogram (gone are the days when only custom-made shirts carried them), get it in the right place. Many Americans have the monograms placed above the breast pocket, but Southerners tend to wear their initials on their sleeve, literally. The European style is on the left side of the shirt, fifth button down. Geeks go for the collar.

Any dress shirt worth its weight in weave will have at least seven buttons. The more buttons, the better it'll be secured in your pants. If you want to show the world that you're a class guy, buy shirts with French cuffs.

The case for custom-made

When it comes to custom-made shirts, the fit should be perfect, so your first concern is fabric. High-quality off-the-rack shirts have yarn counts of sixty to eighty, which means it takes sixty to eighty lengths of thread, each 840 yards long, to equal one pound. The higher the yarn count, the finer the thread, the more expensive the shirt, and the more delicate the material. For the office, a shirt with a yarn count of 140 will make you look like a CEO. Anything over 160 will make you look like a European count. Head Monkeys don't like European counts.

Then comes style. Collars, cuffs, monograms, breast pocket or not—you design your own shirt. A good custom shirtmaker will ask whether you wear a watch, and on which hand, and will then cut that sleeve accordingly. A really good custom shirtmaker will ask to see the watch.

Most shirtmakers require a minimum order of three or four shirts, with each shirt costing $90 and up (way up), depending on yarn count and style. From measurements until delivery usually takes at least three or four weeks.

The difference in price between custom-made and made-to-measure shirts is not that great, so why not splurge? With either, you have the luxury of simply calling your shirtmaker when you want some new shirts and ordering them, assuming you haven't gained more than about ten pounds. Also, the shirtmaker will usually replace those collars and cuffs at a nominal charge (they tend to fray before the body of the shirt).

If you're paying for a custom-made shirt, get a shirt that *looks* custom-made. So forget the breast pocket. A pocketless shirt not only fits better, the lines look cleaner. Go for the French cuffs.

Cleaning

It's best to hand-wash, gently dry, and carefully iron all your dress shirts. It's also best never to feel anger, to be kind to your neighbor, to pray regularly, and to spend weekends ladling out chow at the neighborhood soup kitchen. But let's get real.

You'll probably be sending your shirts out.

The problem with most neighborhood cleaners is that they use high-heat washing machines and industrial-strength presses, both of which shorten your shirt's life. You'll know these places by the heavy creases in your cleaned shirts, the occasional rip, the crushed buttons. Thirty-five to fifty commercial washings (less if you use starch) at most places and that shirt's ready for the rag heap.

If you can find a commercial cleaner that takes a more delicate approach, you're a lucky man. The best way to get lucky is by calling the expensive clothing store in your neighborhood and asking for advice.

If you are the kind of guy who likes to do things right (or you're frugal: most men buy five hundred dress shirts in their life, spending about $20,000, and sending them out for cleaning adds $15,000), then you're ready for the hot stuff.

Use a normal amount of detergent and the gentle wash cycle (to remove perspiration stains, soak the shirt twenty-four hours in salty water before laundering). Throw the shirts in the dryer, but take them out when they're still slightly damp. Fill your iron with some water, then plug it in. Start it on cool and nudge up the heat until you see a little steam.

Do the sleeves and cuffs first, then the shoulders and yoke, then the front and back and collar. Remove plastic stays first. If you don't, their imprint will show. Iron away from any monograms to prevent bunching the fabric around the stitching.

Storage

Hangers.

TIES

Knotted. Around your neck. No wonder guys
have trouble with them.

Length

It should fall to your belt. Slightly below is better than slightly above. And if the thin part of your tie hangs lower than the thick part, you are saying either:

"I am a brilliant scientist/poet/trillionaire, and mere fashion customs are made for others, not me"

or

"I am a *shlub*."

People being who they are, unfortunately, they will probably interpret your look in the latter way.

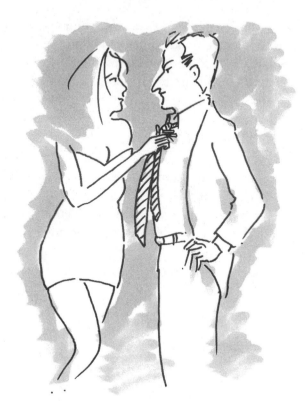

When she says, "Let me straighten that, mein strudel,"
you are not being criticized.

I've found ties that are fifty-four inches, fifty-eight inches, and fifty-six inches. Rather than carrying around a tape measure when you visit your favorite haberdashery (which also makes a rather idiosyncratic statement), wear a tie that fits. Take it off and measure it against a tie you like at the store.

Style

Avoid ties with insignias that symbolize your profession. Avoid ties with pictures of animals. Avoid talking ties, blinking ties, and edible ties. Stick with stripes, solids, and patterns. Wearing a tie with peace symbols can be excused as the eccentricity of a bighearted man with an idiosyncratic sense of style. If you wear dollar signs, you have no excuse.

The knot

There are full Windsor knots, half-Windsor knots, and four-in-hand knots. There's also the yanked-down-to-your-chest-unbuttoned-at-the-collar look, which is great if you want to project a certain impetuous and I'll-pull-your-tongue-out-if-you-cross-me air. Learn one knot (practice in front of a mirror) and stick with it.

Always tie your tie before buttoning the top button of your shirt. After the knot is complete, fold your collar down, then button and make final adjustments. This will save wear and tear on the shirt and tie. You're less likely to choke yourself, too.

The details

To make sure the tie is made properly and will fall correctly, hold the middle over your hand and let the two ends fall. The small end of the tie should fall directly in the center of the large end. Pay attention to the loop on the back of the fat end. If it's made of the same material as the tie, the manufacturer is not skimping on expenses. Also check to see if there's much fusing of the tie—in the lining or between pieces of fabric. If there is, you shouldn't be paying much.

Cleaning

Send it to an establishment that specializes in tie cleaning.

Storage

Never leave a tie knotted when it's not on your body.

SHOES AND SOCKS

Feet on the ground is okay. Head in the clouds can be attractive. Cuffs at the calves is a no-no.

Color

Your shoes should always match the color of your belt. (Your watchband matching either is nice but not necessary.) Your socks are an extension of your suit and, as such, should match your suit, not your shoes.

Even in the most corporate of workplaces, brown shoes are perfectly acceptable with (and in fact can add verve to) gray, blue, and in fact any suit except black.

Style

Unless you wear a lot of classically Italian suits, you should opt for American- or British-style dress shoes, whose substantial heft will complement your clothes. Italian shoes are lighter and more delicate looking. They're what many men call "for wimps."

For the office, stick with black and brown lace-ups. Loafers are too casual for many businesses, and loafers with tassels might say you're ready for a good time, but they don't say you're particularly serious about your job. Cowboy boots are the male equivalent of spike heels.

The details

You can get a pair of shoes for less than $100, but then you'll be getting another pair just like them next year and the year after and the year after that. It makes more sense to spend $300 or more for a pair of sturdy cordovans (the material, not the color) that will last you ten years or more, and which will only cost you the money it takes to get them resoled and shined.

Shop in the afternoon, when your feet are swollen. Insist on having your feet measured separately. And check to make sure the inside of the shoe is leather lined with leather insoles, and that the heel is leather, too. Surfaces should be sewn, not glued.

Buy only over-the-calf socks for work. There are uglier sights than the sight of a man's leg flesh in the office—but none come immediately to mind.

Cleaning

Get regular shines. If your shoes get soaked on a snowy day, stuff them with newspaper to let them dry—slowly, away from heat. Then remove salt stains by sponging the shoes with white vinegar.

Storage

Though conventional wisdom holds that cedar shoe trees are best for absorbing odor and helping maintain the shape of leather shoes, you'd do better with poplar or oak. That's because those woods are harder than cedar and will keep the shoe's shape longer. Just make sure the wood has not been shellacked, so it will soak up sweat and smells. And don't wear the same shoes on consecutive days.

ACCESSORIES

It's the little things that count.

Belts

They should have five holes, the actual length of the belt being measured from the center hole. Make sure stitching and other detailing is well fixed.

Suspenders

Also known as braces, they're functional, masculine, and handsome. Good suit pants are made for button-on suspenders; if not, wear a belt. Do not wear suspenders that perfectly match your socks or tie. It's gimmicky, which is another way of saying cheesy. Clip-on suspenders are beyond cheesy. A belt and suspenders worn at the same time are beyond clip-ons.

Watches

The simpler and less digital, the more elegant. Watches that tell you five time zones, square roots, and when the next lunar eclipse will occur also tell the world that you're kind of strange.

Cuff links

Gold and silver are best. Enamel is fine. Spinning roulette wheels are tacky. Keep them simple.

Wallets, money clips, and key rings

Wallets should be slim and leather and should fit inside your suit's breast pocket. Money clips should be leather or metal and should be used to hold only money, not credit cards or bowling lane receipts. A key ring with more than three or four keys belongs to a man whose life is scattered.

PUTTING IT TOGETHER

Getting beyond the "Honey, what do you think?" approach.

Rule number one: Dress with confidence.
Rule number two: If you find people staring at your clothes, gasping and giggling, maybe you're mistaking low-level insanity, or color blindness, or delusions of grandeur, for confidence. Try another combination next time. Better yet, stick with solid colors.

Rules three through eight: Don't wear a button-down shirt with a double-breasted suit. Don't wear French cuffs with a sport coat or jeans. Don't wear a short-sleeved dress shirt, or if you do, at least get the plastic pocket protector and white socks to complete the look. Don't wear T-shirts underneath anything finer than an oxford cloth. Don't wear running shoes with your suit. Don't go for a "sexy silhouette" look.

The really few other rules: Different shades of the same color look

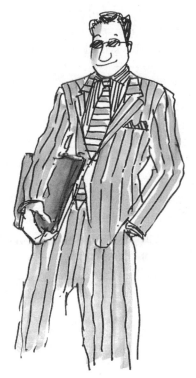

Stripes can *co-exist.*

silly together, unless they're markedly different shades. Stripes can coexist, as long as they're of varying widths. Wear a boldly striped tie with a finely striped shirt, for example. Slender European suits demand long, slender shirt points; full American cuts don't look right with exaggeratedly long shirt points.

TUXEDOS

In the heat of the night.

If you go to at least two or three formal functions a year, buy formal wear. Stick with black and expect to pay at least $600. Some consider a shawl collar old-fashioned. These are the same folks who think watching *It's a Wonderful Life* in black and white is old-fashioned. If you get the shawl collar, wear it only at night. If you're heavy, stay away from the style, as the collar will accentuate the curve of your belly.

Feeling particularly daring? Consider cuffed tuxedo trousers. Now forget them. Most fashion guidelines are made to be bent, broken, and played with. Not this one. The cuffs, originally invented in England, where gentleman farmers strolling around their estates turned up the bottoms of their pants to prevent them from getting soiled, soon spread to tweedy suits and casual suits. Now they're everywhere. Except for formal wear. Keep it that way.

The most elegant tux (or dinner jacket, as it is called by those with trust funds) is not black at all, but midnight blue. Midnight blue actually looks blacker than black at night. Black can take on a sickly green tint under harsh indoor lights.

TOPCOATS

What warms you.

If money is no object, invest in a vicuña garment. It'll set you back maybe as much as $25,000, but it's so soft it makes ordinary cashmere feel like wool. Otherwise, buy wool, cashmere, or camel's hair. The coat should be black, navy, or camel's hair and should fit loosely, sleeves extending slightly below your shirtsleeves, the bottom reaching below your knees. Simple single-breasted, beltless is best; avoid a coat fitted at the waist. You'll be happy after that two-week pizza binge.

The rage the past few years among some forward-thinking fashion plates has been down coats worn over suit coats. This is a trend with all the aesthetic appeal and functionality of the Nehru jacket. Save your down jacket for the wilderness.

BLAZERS

Beyond the prep look. Way beyond.

Start with blue. And don't go any further. The blue blazer could be the single most versatile piece of clothing you ever own. It can dress up a pair of jeans, frame a turtleneck, top off a pair of gray flannel slacks, perfectly complement khakis.

What you want is a classic two-button. The blazer should be made of "doeskin" lightweight wool, which you can wear ten months a year. (You're out of luck in January and August.)

Expect to pay anywhere from $225 to $2,600.

Once you've got this piece, start considering cashmere, and a nice Harris Tweed.

KHAKIS

Eternally cool.

The classic khaki features the flat front, which has, surprise, a flat, pleatless front. Also no cuffs. If you have what those in the fashion industry call a "broad beam," and others call a "lard ass," khakis are available with "full fronts," which still have no pleats, but slightly more room. If you have what those in the fashion industry call a "mutant, Jupiter like, gargantuan beam," forget the classic look and get pleats.

JEANS

Workingman's blues.

Jeans (I know they come in black, brown, white, etc., now) are still best in blue. As honest and American a piece of clothing as you can buy, jeans are also available in a staggering number of styles and makes these days.

Buy jeans a size larger than your usual pants if you're buying the "traditional fit," unless you want to look like a squeezed sausage. If you're looking for a little more room, "relaxed fit" gives you about a half inch more in the seat and knee, and "loose fit" means an extra four inches around the seat and three inches in the thigh.

Ralph Lauren, Tommy Hilfiger, and Calvin Klein make fine jeans. And some of my favorites come from the Gap and Banana Republic. But if you appreciate the roots and iconography of an American classic, stick with Levi's.

Although "stonewashed" used to be strictly for mall girls and guys with gold chains, nowadays all jeans are prewashed, except for original Levi's, which are indigo and feel like canvas.

CLOTHES THAT ARE FINE ALMOST ANYWHERE

They're timeless for a reason.

Polo shirts, turtlenecks, gray flannel slacks, gabardine shirts, wool sweaters, chambray and denim button-down shirts. They look good. They feel good. They are good.

CLOTHES THAT ARE ALSO FINE ALMOST ANYWHERE, AS LONG AS YOU'RE ALONE

"When I became a man, I put away childish things."

Hawaiian shirts, college sweatshirts, hiking shorts with drawstring waistband, T-shirts with messages, sandals with socks, platform shoes, leisure suits. They look funny. They feel funny. They will make winsome blondes say, "Get a life, Lumpy," when you offer to buy them drinks.

ON THE ROAD

A few words about packing and traveling.

You'll need a dopp kit, preferably leather because it lasts, it wears well, and as a fashion editor I know puts it, "it bespeaks a certain elegance." I think this means that if a client happens to use your bathroom, he'll think you're a high roller. But be meticulous, because leather tends to stain.

In the dopp kit, carry a razor, shaving cream, comb, shampoo, deodorant, toothpaste, dental floss, toothbrush, moisturizer, and condoms.

Take two suits if you have more than one business meeting, two or three dress shirts, a couple ties, and one pair of dress shoes. Anything more is foolish. So what if your clothes get dirty? Who cares if you need a suit steamed? What's the difference if you need to buy a brand-spanking-new pair of shoes? If you work for a company that flies you somewhere to do business, you work for a company that will pay for expenses that are absolutely necessary to ensure that you look sharp. If you have any doubts about this (and you *should* have doubts if you think everyone will share your passion for ironed socks), play it safe, hoard meal receipts, and create some phony dinner meetings to cover your cleaning bill.

Also, don't forget a swimming suit, workout clothes, athletic shoes, a sport coat, and if it's cool, a sweater.

If you're like most guys, you'll be carrying your suits and dress shirts in a garment bag. And you'll be worrying about that bag ending up crammed underneath the seat in front of you, rather than resting, nice and neat and flat, in the overhead compartment where it rightfully belongs. So what can you do to gain peace of mind about your defenseless and wrinkle-prone clothes, especially when you're competing with brutish hordes of other guys with garment bags, some of them who actually sink as low as boarding the plane before their aisle is called, which is really tacky?

You can fly first-class, which will purchase legroom *and* a place to hang your garment bag, as well as better food and generally longer-limbed and more beautiful stewar—I mean, flight attendants. But that's expensive.

Or you can invest in an elastic knee brace, available for less than $10 at most sporting goods stores. When the airline representative announces early seating for "first-class passengers and any others needing special assistance," that's your cue to limp up the aisle, dragging that wrapped, sore, and very useful leg of yours. You'll find plenty of room in the overhead compartments. (I know this doesn't sound gentlemanly, sophisticated, or charitable, and I have mixed feelings about even mentioning this elegantly simple if slightly dishonest solution. But these are tough times.)

Do not, once the plane is in flight, do a celebratory cha-cha in the aisle.

GROOMING

You're a naked ape, but you want to be a clean,good-looking naked ape.

Even the best-dressed guy in the world will have the world all to himself if he's unkempt, malodorous, scraggly, repulsive, repellent, frightening, or has a really bad haircut.

Soap and water are a good beginning, but the well-groomed guy needs to know more—about his teeth, his scalp, his digits, his skin. Cleanliness is a necessity. Facials are fey. Here's a map to the middle ground.

The kindest cut

Your haircut is telling the world something. Sometimes that some-thing is "I want to be like Joey Buttafuoco." Other times it's "I refuse to admit that I am aging."

If it's thinning, for God's sake, get it cut. The longer your hair, the thinner it will look. The guys with those hideous comb-overs didn't start out *trying* to look absurd.

How do you find a man who knows his way around a scissors? Eileen Bugnitz, who has styled hair on *Beverly Hills 90210*, among other shows, and who steadfastly refuses to dis Tori Spelling, despite my repeated entreaties, says, "It's like finding a therapist. You have to look for someone you're comfortable with. The best way is through word of mouth. So if you know a guy with a good haircut, ask him."

A good haircut costs $40 and up. Tip about 20 percent, and at least a couple bucks for the person who shampoos your hair.

Keeping it clean

Shampoo. Rinse well. Too much conditioner makes your hair look flat and dull. Use it only a couple days a week.

A New York City hairdresser who charges clients $400 for a haircut suggests dousing your head with apple-cider vinegar. He says it will clean your hair and add a healthy-looking sheen with-out sucking all the natural proteins from your hair, as regular sham-poo sometimes does. I say if you try it, rinse *really* well.

Blow-dryers blow. Avoid them.

Farewell to flakes

Over-the-counter dandruff shampoos with zinc will usually solve the problem if used daily for a week or so. If not, try an over-the-counter tar shampoo (for serious cases only). If that doesn't do the trick, ask your doctor for a prescription for a cleanser containing 2 percent ketoconazole, an antifungal agent proved effective against *Pityrosporum ovale*, a yeast implicated in the problem. Oh, yeah, and buy some light-colored clothes.

If the problem persists, consult a dermatologist.

Going, going, gone

Too much gel does not speed hair loss. Neither does wearing a baseball cap that is too tight, dreaming of bowling balls, or stepping through a metal detector. It's hereditary. Another thing to blame Mom for (though research is pointing the finger at Dad, too). Live with it.

There is one 100 percent effective way to prevent hair loss. It's called castration. I don't recommend it.

The trouble with hairy

As with real estate, sex, and making a pass at your girlfriend's sultry best friend, location is everything.

Where you don't want hair is on your back, in your ears and nostrils, between your eyes. If you have it there, and you're comfortable with yourself and/or are a fabulously wealthy Nobel Prize winner/rock star/software-company CEO, you could care less that you gross some people out. For the rest of you hispid hunks, I'd advise investing in a pair of blunt-tipped scissors and doing spot sprout checks. Nosehair clipping is mandatory. A bush there is gross, and getting rid of it is easy. Ear trims might be more easily performed by a barber. As for the unibrow, it requires tweezers, and some women like it (the brow, not the tweezers). Beastly back? You can get waxed, lasered, or zapped. Or you can keep your shirt on until you find someone who loves you up front.

Shaving

In ancient Rome, young men sacrificed their first beard to the gods. During the Middle Ages, the Church denied communion to men who weren't clean-shaven. And though a beard had long been a symbol of sexual prowess, when Alexander the Great, worried about large numbers of his foot soldiers being offed in battle, rode to the top of a mountain one day and sat there watching his enemies grab his soldier's beards, lift them, and slit their throat, he ordered his army to shave every day.

Shaving is still about sex, and masculinity and social control, as well as vanity, as the daily removal of dead skin makes a man look good as well as feel young. All those factors help explain why 86 million Americans fifteen and older peer into mirrors as often as six times a week while they apply cold steel to their warm flesh.

If you're one of them, here are some ways to avoid the cruelest cuts:

If you're a blade man (about 70 percent of you are), shave after you shower. The hot water and steam soften your beard. (A new generation of fog-proof mirrors makes shaving while you shower a viable alternative.)

When you're lathered and ready, start at the sideburns and make short strokes in the direction of your beard's growth. The neck follows the cheeks, and the upper lip and chin come last. That's because whiskers there are the thickest and you want to give them the most time to soften up under all the foam.

Once you're done, don't forget to wash. That fresh feeling you created doesn't come from just being newly hairless. It's because you've just removed an entire layer of dead skin. The bad news is, you've just spread a bunch of bacteria around your kisser. So wash up. And slap on some aftershave. No, no, not the stuff that feels like battery acid and smells like eau de Adman. That's the old-fashioned, alcohol-based stuff that tightens your pores and dries out your skin. These days, aftershave is all about moisturizing and healing, rather than "stings like hell." Even the products that contain alcohol also usually have moisturizer.

If you're one of the 10 percent of American men who suffer from razor burn, and you can't face the prospect of a beard, be gentle. Easy does it. If the shave isn't close enough for your taste, try shaving twice, but gently. On days when the burn is really bad, buy an over-the-counter ointment with 1 percent hydro-cortisone.

If you have curly hair or are just plain unlucky, one of your recently barbered facial hairs might decide to turn back into your skin instead of growing out again. To avoid those painful (some-times infected) pustules, your best bet is to grow a beard. If you can't do that, you can try a depilatory cream, which chemically dissolves hair off at the surface level. But that can aggravate sensi-tive skin. Then there's electrolysis. It hurts. It costs. It's final.

Saving face

Your skin is an organ. It is dying. The world is becoming a more cruel place, what with global warming, a depleting ozone layer, and offices with no windows and clouds of nasty organisms floating around. Get the picture?

Your face is probably flaking right now. So put some moisturizer on. It won't kill you. In fact, it will make you feel better, look younger, and will keep wrinkles away for a little while. At the very least, use the stuff when flying. (And remember to drink extra water, too.)

If you're really worried about wrinkles, you could try alphahy-droxy acid or fruit acids, or the newly available vitamin C com-pounds that cost $75 an ounce. You could also get plastic surgery. On the other hand, some of my good friends are dermatologists and plastic surgeons, but what's wrong with wrinkles?

Digitally correct

Consider the advice from fashion and grooming experts who promise that hanging cuticles and nonbuffed nails will cost you contracts and generally leach love and truth from your life. Now laugh out loud.

Keep your nails short and keep 'em clean. Other than that, do you really care what a guy's fingernails look like? If you want a manicure, it won't hurt. (Actually it feels pretty good.) But pass on the polish. Strictly for guys with pinky rings and fat stogies. Pedicure? Puh-leeze.

Reality bites

You might think that it's normal to lose a tooth or two as you age. You might also think that you can get mercury poisoning from silver amalgam fillings and that root canal is the yardstick by which all other pain is measured.

If so, you are wrong, wrong, wrong, Smiley. You get more mercury from eating one fish than from walking around with a silver amalgam filling your entire life. Root canal can be quite literally painless. And the only reason for you to lose any of your choppers is through ignorance and sloth.

To prevent tooth decay, brush twice a day, floss every night, and visit your dentist twice a year. When you brush, do so for three minutes (get an egg timer), and make tight, tiny circles while holding your toothbrush at a forty-five-degree angle just at the gum line. Don't use a back-and-forth sawing motion. Stick with a soft—not hard—bristle.

To avoid nasty bacteria, replace your toothbrush every month. To avoid losing a chopper or two to accident, don't chew ice or unpopped popcorn kernels or play contact sports without a mouth guard.

And remember: Electric toothbrushes are cool, but unnecessary; baking soda has absolutely no value other than as a marketing tool; and one in four men will suffer from gum disease. This comes from bad dental hygiene, a too-hard brush, and the genetic crapshoot. If caught early, in the gingivitis stage, it often requires nothing more than increased vigilance in brushing.

Also, unsupervised home bleaching can work. It can also not work. If you want whiter teeth, ask your dentist to do it for you. He'll make a custom-fitted mouthpiece to keep the potent peroxide gel on your enamel and off your gums. It should cost about $300 and take four to six weeks.

Our bodies, our smells

Lesson One: Female voles don't even bother to ovulate if they don't smell a studly little male vole nearby who might mate with them, and when a female pig in estrus smells a certain chemical produced by the boar, she reflexively begins a stiff-legged mating dance.

Lesson Two: Beyond all the "citrus notes" and "masculine scents" that cologne companies babble on about, none of them have yet captured the pheromone responsible for driving women wild with lust. (For that, you'll need things like humor, wisdom, money, and a nice car.)

Lesson Three: You produce certain smells, thanks to your apocrine glands located near the armpits and genitals. When those

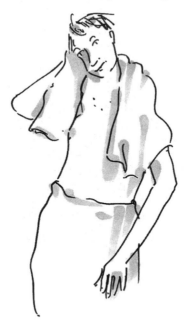

Moral: Wash well.

smells combine with bacteria trapped under clothes all day, the smells definitely don't attract anyone.

Moral: Wash well. Use an antibacterial soap for good measure. If you're a heavy sweater, try an antiperspirant containing aluminum zirconium. If that doesn't work, see a doctor.

And if you're going to use cologne, remember that less is more.

Breathtaking

When colleagues are running at your approach and the deli-counter guy is swooning at your order, it might mean nothing more sinister than a diet a little too heavy in garlic, onion, and liverwurst. Then again, bad breath might be a sign of diabetes, cancer, or a bacterial infestation of the inside of your mouth.

First, try brushing (tongue, too) and flossing more frequently, cutting down on the more repugnant-smelling foods, eating an apple occasionally to get the saliva flowing. If the odor doesn't abate, see a dentist. You might have a gum disease or worse.

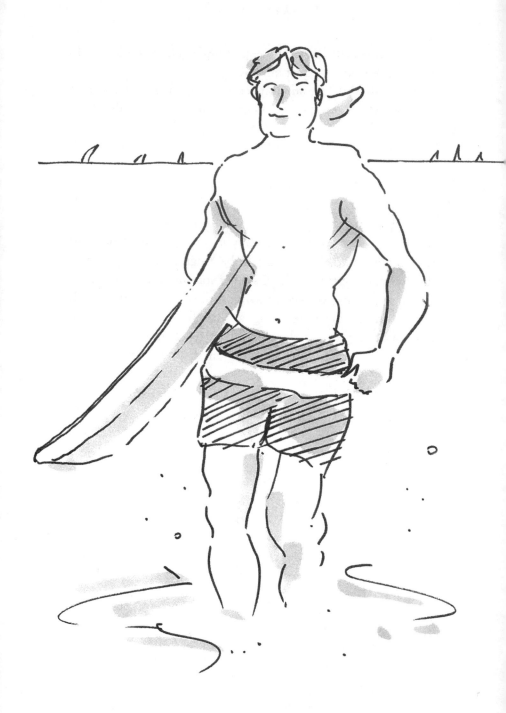

FEELING STRONG

THE BOTTOM LINE

Exercise, eat your vegetables, don't smoke, and get plenty of rest. And drink lots of water.

INDISPENSABLE ITEMS

Gym clothes, cross-training shoes, a set of dumbbells or a gym membership.

COMMON QUESTIONS

Should I take vitamin supplements? How often should I have a prostate exam? Am I really better off drinking two glasses of wine than abstaining from alcohol completely? How much fat should be in my diet? How do I lose love handles? How much sleep do I really need? Would I be better off quitting coffee?

Pasta makes you fat!

Running guru dies while jogging!

Detecting prostate cancer early doesn't increase your chances of living longer!

Too many vitamins can kill ya!

Your sperm are dying!!!

Food "experts" can't agree on a thing, and the one you saw last night on the infomercial is kind of creepy, anyway!

Pay close attention to every health headline and nutrition news-flash coming your way, and no one would blame you for giving up, grabbing a steak (rare) and Scotch (neat) and lumbering quietly into the land of lard and lassitude. The problem with that kind of attitude (in addition to its leading inevitably to a more than passing resemblance to Jabba the Hut) is that it's based on bad information.

While the headlines aren't exactly *wrong,* they're misleading. That's because newspapers and magazines take complicated research, boil it down to a flashy couple of sentences, ignore the context in which the experiment took place, then slap a frighten-ing summary on top.

What you need is context, and a few general principles to help you. You need to know what to eat, how to exercise, what vitamins and drugs you should take, which ones you should avoid. You need to know about sex and disease and aging. You need to know what will make you feel strong and live long.

Above all, you need to know that physical fitness means more than rippling abs and bulging biceps. It means more energy, better sex, deeper sleep, higher-quality serenity—exactly what a carefully ingested combination of methamphetamines, barbiturates, Prozac, and cocaine would give you, except you would die quickly, and besides, it would also cost a lot more and your friends and family would disapprove.

EXERCISE

Move it.

***Reasons to avoid regularly doing
something that involves
sweating and breathing hard***

You have to sweat and breathe hard.

You don't have time.

It might not help you live any longer, anyway.

Seinfeld's on tonight and you don't know how to work your VCR, and besides, isn't your value as a human being based on more than how you look in a tank top, I mean, *Jesus*, what about my mind, my soul, my *being!*

***Reasons you should adopt a regular
exercise program***

It will lower your risk of coronary artery disease, adult-onset diabetes, and the likelihood of certain cancers.

It will reduce high blood pressure.

It will reduce cholesterol levels.

It will delay the onset of osteoporosis.

It will decrease anxiety and tension, increase happiness and creativity, and help you sleep better.

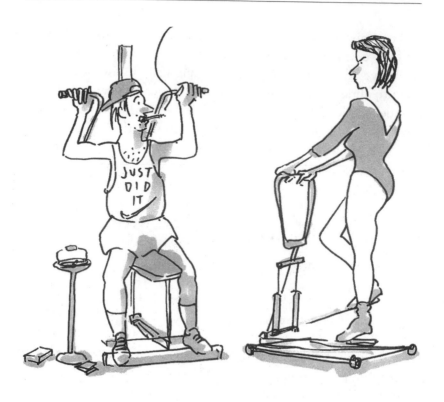

Women who exercise like men who exercise.

It will make you look better.

Women who exercise like men who exercise.

Do you really want to be one of the guys whom the marketing weasels at clothing companies are thinking about when they devise phrases like "loose fit" and "mature shape"?

That chunk of blueberry pie with vanilla ice cream? Why the hell not? You'll work it off later.

How hard you need to work out
to reap the benefits

At a level in which you are breathing hard but can still carry on a conversation. To be more precise, subtract your age in years from

220. That's your maximum heart rate, and if you're thirty-five, it's 185. Experts generally recommend that healthy adults work out in the 60 to 85 percent target heart-rate range to achieve maximum fat-burning, happy-chemical-producing benefits. So, if you're thirty-five, that's 185 × .60 and 185 × .80, which equals a heart rate range of 111 to 148. (For those who are obese or mega couch potatoes with a low baseline fitness level, working out at 40 to 60 percent is suggested to start.)

And how often?

At least twenty minutes at least three or four times a week. Longer and harder and the benefits are more dramatic.

And what's going on in there?

If you're breathing hard but steadily, you're doing aerobic ("with air") exercise. Aerobic workouts transform your body by first transforming the fibers in your muscles. They become more effective at absorbing oxygen and nutrients from the bloodstream to use as fuel. They also better oxidize fats and carbohydrates, which is why you lose weight. Meanwhile, your lungs get more efficient (you breathe deeply and less frequently) and your heart becomes stronger, pushing more blood with each heartbeat. This enables it to pump less frequently, which makes for a lot less wear and tear on the heart muscle.

And as for living longer

You'll need to burn at least fifteen hundred calories a week, which means you need to jog or walk really fast about fifteen miles a week.

Getting started

You could check around town to see where your most fetching local TV newsanchor works out, because you've always wanted to see her sweaty. You could spend a few hours on the phone, calling health clubs and asking what percentage of their staff members hold degrees and certifications from the American College of Sports Medicine (ACSM), the American Council on Exercise (ACE), or the Aerobics and Fitness Association in America (AFAA). You could send a self-addressed, stamped envelope to the International Association of Fitness Professionals. They provide excellent free pamphlets on how to start a fitness program, how to choose a quality fitness facility, a personal trainer, or an aerobics instructor and class that's right for you.

Then again, you could simply *get your fat butt up and just get started, you miserable blob of Jell-O*. (Sorry, but sometimes guys need to hear that.)

Put on some sneakers and walk fast for twenty minutes. Pump your arms. Breathe hard. Repeat the day after tomorrow. Keep repeating until no one's calling you a fat blob of Jell-O.

Oh, yeah, if it's been years, if you're over forty and/or if your family has a history of heart disease, see a doctor first.

Staying with it

After a couple of weeks, you'll notice more energy, less fatigue, a greater sense of well-being. Your clothes will fit better. You need more encouragement than that?

Cooling down

If you come to a dead halt after vigorous exercise—whether you get stuck at a stoplight in the middle of your run, stand motionless while you take your pulse, or stop and get distracted chatting with friends—your blood pressure will drop, but your heart will still be beating furiously. Blood can pool in certain parts of the body, limiting the amount getting back up to the heart and brain, and this can lead to light-headedness, injury to the heart muscle, or even sudden death. There is widespread agreement among exercise physiologists that this is not a good thing.

Stretching

There's no reason to stretch before or after exercise, if you don't mind soreness, chronic and acute pain, and possibly serious injury. If you want to avoid those things, stretch.

Warm up for a few minutes before you stretch. Jog in place for a short time. Or pedal lightly. This gets your muscles warm and slightly limber. Stretching cold, tight muscles hurts. It might also mean a pulled muscle.

After your workout, and after you've cooled down, stretch. Don't bounce or jerk. Move slowly into each stretch, sustain it, and sense how your muscles *feel*. Don't hold your breath, but breathe slowly with each stretch. A basic stretch for any exercise involving your legs is to sit on the floor with your legs spread. Bend as far over each leg as possible, alternating legs. Hold each stretch for about fifteen seconds. Repeat at least three times.

The heavy stuff

While aerobic exercise makes you happy and healthy, adding resistance training to your workout makes you happy and healthy and ripped. You're stressing your musculoskeletal system beyond its normal capacity. You're causing tiny tears in your muscles, then creating new tissue to heal over the tears, which increases the mass of the muscle. You're building bulging biceps, washboard abs, ripped and supercut legs and chest and less fat, which means that your metabolism will run faster, so you'll be burning more calories just standing around than you would had you never picked up that dumbbell.

Translation: Babes.

Now, you've no doubt encountered men for whom the term *musclehead* is an all-too-apt moniker, considering their freakishly developed chests and biceps and spindly legs. The sad thing is, not only are these gorillas creating cartoonishly lumpy shapes, they're also increasing their chance of injury. What you want is balance.

So learn the opposing muscle groups. Biceps-triceps. Chest-back. Hamstrings-quadriceps. Work the large-muscle groups before the smaller ones. Never work out the same muscle group two days in a row, because then it won't have time to heal.

Each weight-lifting exercise should consist of ten to fifteen repetitions, and you should repeat the set three times. If you can lift a weight with ease fifteen times, it's too light. If you can't do ten reps, it's too heavy. You'll probably start on machines, because free weights require more work from your muscles to hold them in the correct position and prevent any tipping from side to side. Once you have developed some minimal strength, though, you'll want to move to the free weights, *because* they demand more of your muscles. Also, as many guys in the gym so elegantly put it, "machines are for girls."

Whatever exercise you're doing, use proper form. That means if you're doing biceps curls, don't use your shoulders. Bench presses? Don't arch your back. If you're lifting weights in a gym, get a staff member to help you develop a regimen you can follow. If you're working out at home, hire a personal trainer to help you get started.

If you never touch a weight, use these simple exercises:

Push-ups—for the chest and triceps.

Pull-ups—for the back and biceps.

Lifting heavy objects over your head—for the shoulders.

Running, biking, walking—for the legs.

Pain

Soreness is good. It means you're breaking down the microfibers in your muscles, which will lead to bigger, stronger muscles. Sharp, stabbing pain is not good. Lay off the weights and see a doctor.

What's the minimum requirement?

Two to three sets per body part, twice a week. You'll see changes within your first two weeks.

THE BELLY OF THE BEAST

Getting to the gut of things.

You are paying too much attention to your
abdominal muscles if

You call them abs.

You own an entire book dedicated to them.

You check out other guys' abs.

You spend a lot of time marveling at the exquisite craftsmanship and heartrending beauty of the Abdominizer.

You have been known to raise your shirt and say, "Check out my six-pack."

You are paying too little attention to your
abdominal muscles if

You haven't seen your toes in a while.

The owner of your business always asks you to play Santa at the holiday party, even though he knows you're Jewish.

You loosen your belt at least twice a week and exclaim, "Oh, baby, now that's good eating."

People refer to your stomach as "the labonza," "the old bread basket," "the chicken cemetery," "the bay window," or "the front porch."

Small children ask if you're pregnant.

You are paying the wrong type of attention
to your abdominal muscles if

You are fond of quoting Cato the Elder, who said, "It is a hard matter, my fellow citizens, to argue with the belly, since it has no ears."

When you approach the dinner table, you grab two handfuls of flesh and recite a poem fragment from Delmore Schwartz, who wrote "that inescapable animal walks with me / . . . A caricature, a swollen shadow / or stupid clown of the spirit's motive . . ."

You refer to your stomach in the third person, and as a demanding creature, as in: "Ozzie is hungry. Ozzie must feed. I must obey."

Before a nation turned its weary eyes to male midsections, the abdominal muscles were responsible for simple things—like helping balance, increasing athletic performance, improving posture, supporting the lower back, providing a big lift during sexual intercourse. The more fit they were, the better off you were, in nearly any position in which you found yourself.

Now, of course, abs aren't abs unless they're ripped, rippling, washboard, and cut. I personally have nothing against the lean and hungry look, but really, isn't this obsession with a man's middle just a little bizarre?

Luckily, the following regimen, designed to create better-functioning abdominals, will also make them better looking. You can work the abs every day. Warning: Unless you eat right and regularly burn fat with aerobic exercise, you'll still be playing St. Nick. Spot reduction does not work. To lose the love handles, you still have to cut the fat.

The basic crunch

Lie on your back, knees bent, feet flat on the floor, your back in its natural (slightly curved) position. Place hands behind your head, elbows out to the sides. Take a deep breath, then exhale as you flatten your lower back into the floor and raise your shoulder blades just a few inches off the ground. Lift with your abs, not your neck—you should be eyeing the ceiling, head aligned with your spine. Imagine being lifted by someone above you who is pulling a string attached to your chest. Hold two seconds, then slowly lower to start position. Try for one set of ten to twenty reps, eventually working up to three sets with one-minute breaks in between.

The crossover crunch

This works the obliques that run diagonally along the sides of your body. It's performed the same as the basic crunch, except when raising the shoulder up off the floor, imagine the right shoulder being pulled like a magnet in the direction of your left knee, then left shoulder to right knee.

The reverse crunch

Lie on your back, legs raised so thighs are perpendicular to the floor, knees bent at around a ninety-degree angle, and use the lower abs to raise your hips off the floor a few inches, knees heading in the direction of your forehead. Hold a few seconds and release. This works the transversus abdominis, which sits underneath your other abdominal muscles and connects low on the pubic bone.

SEX

Maybe the brain is the most important organ. Then again, it's nice to have everything else in working order.

Great sex is about sharing, and communication and intimacy. It's about love. A focus on the purely physical aspects of what should be a spiritual experience is sadly shortsighted. And a man preoccupied with such things as aphrodisiacs and erections and how his equipment changes as he gets older, well, that man is looking in the flesh for what is more appropriately found in the soul. That man is doomed. That man deserves pity.

Now that we all feel better, let's talk about things like aphrodisiacs and erections and how your equipment changes as you get older.

Aphrodisiacs

Injected directly into the penis, a few milligrams of papaverine will give you an almost instant, rock-hard erection (as demonstrated quite dramatically by a scientist who did just that at a Las Vegas convention of urologists in 1983; he stepped from behind the podium, unzipped his pants, then wandered among the assembled penis doctors).

The problem is, sticking a needle into your penis is not exactly a mood enhancer (though Israeli scientists are working on a topical solution). That's just one reason why men wanting faster and stronger erections are trying testosterone supplements (available only by prescription) and yohimbe, which is carried in health-food stores. Both carry unpleasant and dangerous side effects, including dizziness, the shakes, increased risk of stroke and prostate disease. Oh, yeah, and papaverine users have reported priapism—an unending and painful erection that might land you in an emergency room. In extreme cases, the penis has to be cut to relieve the swelling. Might I suggest a nice chardonnay instead to set the mood?

Masturbation

And speaking of sex that has nothing to do with communing with another human being, masturbation still remains a taboo subject, a topic that gets politicians such as Joycelyn Elders relieved from duty just for mentioning it, and celebrities such as Pee-wee Herman shunned for doing it. (Although he probably should have picked a better place than a movie theater.)

Yet despite all the shame and guilt that has been heaped on the practice (it has been condemned by Chistianity and Judaism for centuries), it is, I'm guessing, not entirely unknown to you.

Why make friends with five-fingered Rosy? Every time you ejaculate, it flushes the system, sending blood and oxygen coursing through the vascular system and nourishing tissues; regular workouts like this are necessary to keep the penis flexible, muscles toned, fluid pathways clear, and you ready for action well into the golden years. And, just in case you're wondering, urologist James Mulcahy, M.D., assures us these benefits are gained whether one utilizes the penis for intercourse or a solo performance: "Your body won't know the difference."

How your equipment changes as you age

Gone are the days when your biggest concern was pepperoni versus mushroom. Now you have to worry about your career, your finances, maybe even your marital and parental problems. Is it any wonder as you head into your thirties or forties, and age is already working its inevitable magic on your body, that it's tougher to get and maintain erections? It shouldn't be. But it is. And that's why so many guys end up in their doctor's office, asking about impotence when it is merely aging at work.

Things to lament

It takes longer to get an erection, and it takes longer between erections. Between ages forty-five and fifty-five, the period between "ejaculatory inevitability" (the point of no return) and emission becomes briefer. Eventually, this two-stage aspect of a young man's orgasm becomes one shorter orgasmic reflex. Inevitably, your ejaculations become less powerful, explosive, and yes, enjoyable.

Thing to rejoice about

You don't come as quickly.

Another thing to rejoice about

You're more secure in who you are, wealthier, wiser, maybe even healthier than you used to be, and consequently sexier.

When the spirit's willing, but the flesh . . .

Defined by some as within a minute of penetration, by others as within eight thrusts, premature ejaculation is probably best summed up by the American Psychiatric Association, which defines it as "occurring before the individual wishes it."

Here's a trick to stop it, called the squeeze technique. Place your thumb on the back and index finger on the front of the penis midshaft, just under the head, and squeeze firmly for fifteen seconds while relaxing the muscles in your butt and legs. Wait about thirty seconds before resuming stimulation. This may need to be repeated four or five times in one session, but with experience, the ability will become automatic.

Impotence

It's not occasional failure. It's not being too tired to perform. What it is, clinically speaking, is this: When you can't have an erection adequate for penetration and/or cannot sustain it long enough to reach orgasm in at least 75 percent of attempts at intercourse. Erection problems affect about 10 million men, and sex therapists boast a success rate of 60 to 80 percent, depending on the cause.

If you have an erection when you're sleeping (a lab can tell you), your problem is psychological or emotional, not physical.

Physical factors might include sleeping pills, alcohol, diuretics, high-blood-pressure and heart-disease medications, tranquilizers or antidepressants (if taken for long periods or the dose is too high), fatigue, hormonal imbalances, and prostate infections.

Often, adjusting medication solves the problem. When underlying physical factors cannot be taken care of, doctors suggest implants and vacuum erection devices and various pumps. Ask your doctor.

By the numbers

Average number of orgasms (including solo) per year, according to Clyde E. Martin, Ph.D., former researcher at the labs of the National Institute on Aging, Baltimore

AGE	ORGASMS
20	104
30	121
40	84
50	52
60	35
70	22

Average number of erections per night when
sleeping, according to studies by researchers at
Eastern Virginia Medical School and Baylor
College of Medicine

AGE	NUMBER	TOTAL TIME ERECT (IN MINUTES)
Under 40	4.20	141.0
40–49	3.90	134.0
50–59	3.65	127.5
60 and over	3.60	109.5

Angles of erection, according to researcher
Clyde E. Martin, Ph.D., who also wrote the seminal
(no pun intended) Sexual Behavior in the
Human Male

AGE	ANGLE (WHEN STANDING)
20	10 DEGREES ABOVE HORIZONTAL
30	20 DEGREES ABOVE HORIZONTAL
40	SLIGHTLY ABOVE HORIZONTAL
50	SLIGHTLY BELOW HORIZONTAL
70	25 DEGREES BELOW HORIZONTAL

YOUR BODY, AN OWNER'S MANUAL

It's yours, and yours only. Learn its secrets.

Hair

If you've got red hair, there are an average of 80,000 hairs on your head; brown, 100,000; blond, 120,000. You're losing about 50 to 100 hairs a day, and if you're like 42 million other guys in the United States, it's falling out faster than it's growing in.

The upshot: Live with it. Rogaine manufacturers must solemnly note that hair growth varies from person to person and for many the drug only produces thin, fine hairs, and for others, nothing at all. And hair plugs look like just that—little sprigs of hair sticking straight up out of your head like a Chia Pet. Hey, look around—basketball's Michael Jordan and *Star Trek*'s Patrick Stewart are just two eminently cool and popular cult figures who prove that when it comes to looks, locks are in no way a prerequisite.

Brain

Like your parts farther south, use it or lose it, pal. "Doing mentally stimulating activities may help keep more brain cells alive as well as preserve the connections between them," says Marilyn Albert, M.D., associate professor of psychiatry and neurology at Harvard Medical School. Research has even shown that the more you exercise the mind, the better the rest of your parts can be. Pianists who were only allowed to practice a music selection in their head were just as adept at playing it as those who had really practiced; women who imagined doing quadriceps exercises instead of actually moving the leg saw strength gains (albeit small ones) and muscle improvement.

The upshot: Read, write letters, do the crossword, buy a hand-held video game, daydream on the subway home, sing songs in your head, do whatever you want (besides sitting around like a slug in front of the TV) to keep that mind active.

Skin

Yes, it is the largest organ in the body and would cover, well, if you were filleted, about two square yards and weigh more than ten pounds. And while skin and sun are a great team in terms of producing vitamin D (an essential nutrient for healthy bones and one of the few our body can manufacture on its own), the risks of unprotected exposure to the sun are great, and ever on the increase. Besides the visible effects of aging—dry, wrinkled, thickened, and leathery skin—overexposure to the sun is also responsible for the more serious skin cancer, melanoma, which will attack nearly 22,000 men this year and kill about 4,600. Pay attention to the early warning signs by monitoring moles and freckles with the ABCD system: Look for *asymmetry* (one half of a mole different from the other half); *border irregularity* (edges are ragged, notched, blurred); *color* (uneven pigmentation); and *diameter* (greater than 6 mm or any sudden grown in size).

The upshot: Wear sunscreen with a sun protection factor (SPF) of at least 15 *every day*, applied a half hour before you go out, if possible. Pick up a scent-free, sunscreen-enriched moisturizer for the face, which will defend your face from the daily assaults of ultraviolet rays (which pierce clouds, by the way, and can affect you even on gray days) and will also fend off the appearance of fine lines and wrinkles, making you look younger and more vital for longer than a tan could ever do. A wide-brimmed hat, which handily deflects some rays from the face, wouldn't hurt either.

Heart

The major problem with heart disease is that it happens with little or no warning. Some men have signs of coronary insufficiency, e.g., chest discomfort, shortness of breath, sweating, or lightheadedness, but frequently no major symptoms arise. As physician and author Stephen T. Sinatra notes, it is "ominous in its silence."

The upshot: Take an aspirin daily, if your doctor thinks you would benefit from it; studies have shown such a regimen, some-

THE GENTLEMAN'S GUIDE TO LIFE

times with less than the dosage in a typical tablet, can significantly reduce your risk of heart attack. But there are lots of other heart-healthy possibilities, too: Get a pet, keep in touch with friends, try a yoga, meditation, or tai chi class, learn how to deal with recurring feelings of hostility and rage, walk around the block each evening. All these things have been shown to reduce cardiovascular disease risk and to complement the basics that everyone knows: Eat right (keeping fat to under 20 percent of overall calories), exercise, drop those unnecessary extra pounds, monitor your various cholesterol levels, and *quit smoking*.

Lungs

Ever notice how people act when they're under a tight deadline? "They run around sighing, trying to dump tension so they can be fully present to get the job done," says Dan Howard, spiritual awareness coordinator (yeah, if you had a title like that, you'd be breathing easy, too) at Canyon Ranch in the Berkshires.

The upshot: Learn to breathe fully, deeply. By taking a few moments when you're stressed, or prophylactically, say, every day on your way in to work, you will not only optimize the amount of oxygen taken in by the body and delivered to tissues and cells, but also be calmer and more alert. Try this exercise: Breathe in deep through the nose, and instead of raising shoulders up and down, let the breath fill you, expanding your diaphragm and pushing out your stomach so that you feel as if a balloon under each arm were slowly being filled with air, slightly lifting them. Then exhale, allowing the stomach to return inward. Breathe in for a count of four, hold for a moment and relax, then exhale for a count of eight, holding and relaxing at the very end of your breath. Repeat as many times as you want.

Testicles

Those sperm- and testosterone-producing balls of yours are full of delicately coiled tubules from which sperm is secreted. These wonders of gravity and balance have a nasty habit of picking up cancer early in a man's career—often in one's twenties. In fact, it is one of the most common cancers in men aged fifteen to thirty-four. If discovered in its early stages, however, it can be treated promptly and effectively. The first symptoms include an enlarged testicle and a change in its consistency, often accompanied by a dull ache.

The upshot: Testicular self-exam, once a month, in the shower (where warm water induces the testes to descend a bit farther from the body). Roll each testicle between both thumbs and forefingers, feeling for bumps and lumps. Anything that breaks the smooth flow—consult your doctor.

Legs

Are you even? Too often when working out, we play up one muscle at the expense of its partner—we do curl after curl to get big biceps and forget about triceps extensions. Same with the legs. People emphasize the quads and disregard the hamstrings.

The upshot: Make sure to do quad *and* hamstring exercises. That way, you'll keep your knee properly stabilized and will help absorb stresses that normally shoot to the knee when running, playing tennis, or participating in any impact activity. It will also help strengthen the knee for pivot sports such as racquetball, basketball, touch football, where the risk of tearing or rupturing the anterior cruciate ligament (ACL, a major knee support) is great.

Feet

It's called tinea pedis, athlete's foot to you and me. A common skin condition where previously harmless fungi, given the opportunity to stretch out in a moist or sweaty environment down in your shoes, cause scaling, itching, and redness on the soles and between the toes. Though commonly believed to be contagious, it's actually unlikely that you'll pick it up from a barefoot stroll across the locker-room floor.

The upshot: Wash your feet daily, dry them *thoroughly* (remember between toes), wear cotton (not synthetic) socks and change them if they get damp. To relax your feet after a day of hiking, one-on-one basketball, or just tramping through the nine-to-five concrete jungle (they sustain 5 million pounds of impact each day), try a simple foot massage.

THINGS YOU SHOULD STOP DOING TO LIVE LONGER AND FEEL BETTER

When? Now.

Smoking

It hurts your heart, your lungs, your skin. It increases the chances of all sorts of diseases. Plus, it stinks.

Drinking alcohol

Yeah, I know about the studies showing that a couple of glasses of wine a day might cut your risk of heart disease. But so will eating vegetables and working out. And broccoli and free weights won't shrink brain tissue, cause pancreatic and intestinal disorders, rot your liver, raise your blood pressure, disturb your sleep, dampen your sexual performance, shut down your sperm production, interfere with the body's absorption of vitamins and minerals . . . well, you get the idea.

Weighing Yourself

What's the point of constantly weighing yourself when it only gets you down? Your body weight fluctuates from day to day, but overly conscientious dieters are usually way too swayed by the scale and freak out as soon as it starts creeping up a few points. Some 70 percent of dieters weigh themselves once a week, reports an FDA survey, but diet experts say hopping on the scale once every two weeks is plenty. "Virtually every fat person has a scale, so it's a safe bet that scales don't keep people thin," says Stephen P. Gullo,

Ph.D., a diet expert and author of *Thin Tastes Better*. Besides, muscle weighs more than fat, anyway. It makes more sense to pay
attention to how your clothes fit.

Skipping meals

When the body is deprived of food, even for a short time, it slows
metabolism and burns fat less quickly, as it used to do in the good
old days when we had to track down a gazelle for dinner. Sumo
wrestlers skip breakfast. Think about it over oatmeal.

Touching your feet before your privates

Scratching your feet, clipping toenails, or otherwise grooming the
feet, then touching the genital area, can transfer yeast infections
from foot to groin, which can lead to jock itch.

THINGS YOU SHOULD START DOING TO
LIVE LONGER AND FEEL BETTER

Same time frame as above.

Cleaning up your barbecue manners

Would you dip a hamburger in the sump behind your house before
you served it to your guests? And yet how often do you use the
same plate to bring out the raw hamburger meat from the refriger-
ator and later deliver the cooked burgers to the table and your
guests? Well, the juices on that plate from the raw meat may not
hold as many microbes and bacteria as your backyard sump, but
they can do just as much damage. As if the runs aren't bad enough,
food poisoning kills up to nine thousand people a year (the elderly,
pregnant women, and those with compromised immune systems
are especially vulnerable). So serve cooked foods on clean dishes,
clean cutting boards of raw-meat juices before using them to chop

up salads or other foods that won't be cooked, thoroughly cook all food till juices run clear (not red or pink).

Drinking up

Water, that is. It helps us regulate body temperature, maintain blood volume, and remove wastes from the body. Eight glasses a day at least. More if you're working out.

Ordering special meals when you make plane reservations

Most major carriers offer a wide range of alternative fare, from low-fat to kosher to vegetarian. Because it has to be specially prepared, the food is usually fresher, healthier, and tastes better.

Letting go of a grudge

No matter how egregious the slight, no matter how justified your feelings of ill will may be, holding a grudge is more likely to harm you than the person who committed the offense. Not only does it waste time and energy, but the hostility that you maintain can contribute to heart disease, ulcers, and other physical ailments.

Standing up straight

Your mom may not have known this when she bugged you about it as a kid, but good posture can add inches to your height, conceal the bulge in the belly, help prevent chronic back pain, and make you look tougher.

Laughing

It not only feels good, it does the body good. Laughter researchers (yes, there are such things) have determined that when we laugh, respiration and circulation are enhanced and internal organs are massaged by the physical movement of our body. It's been called "inner jogging." New research suggests laughter may also have some effect on stress-related hormones and T-cell activity.

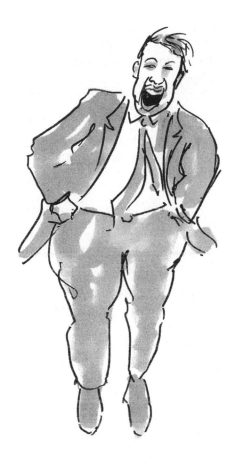

Inner jogging.

EAT!

You are a machine. So fuel up.

Do you *really* think a diet of cheeseburgers, fries, and beer is going to kill you? Do you truly believe the naysayers and antipleasure zealots who think *taste* is a four-letter word? Can you see yourself, a manly man, actually eating something called tofu?

No, no, and no, right?

Well, right, if the prospect of early death doesn't faze you, not to mention the years you do have left being marked by sluggishness, disease, and all around feeling like a lump of blubber.

Too much cholesterol can lead to such problems as arteriosclerosis, heart disease, hypertension, and diabetes, to name a few. Cancer? Doctors say one-third of it in men is linked to diet.

That doesn't mean you have to give up meat. It does mean you should use your head when you're feeding your face.

What to eat

First off, cut the fat. The government recommends that you keep fat to 30 percent or less of your total caloric intake. Dr. Dean Ornish suggests 10 percent as a better number. Ornish has proven that his diet, combined with exercise and meditation, can not only prevent heart disease, but can actually reverse it. So whom are you going to trust, him or the government?

And while you're keeping the fat down, keep the animal fat way down. That's the stuff that's been implicated in heart attacks and artery clogging. So pass on the butter and avoid the steak. Go for fish and vegetables instead. You're shooting for 10 to 20 percent fat, about 20 percent protein, and 60 percent carbohydrates. What can you eat? Fruits, vegetables, rice and beans, egg whites, skim milk. And don't forget the water.

A healthy diet is heaviest in grain-based foods, rich in complex carbs, and lightest in fats, oils, and sweets. The U.S. Department of Agriculture recommends a daily diet of

6–11 servings: bread, cereal, rice, pasta
3–5 servings: vegetables
2–4 servings: fruit
2–3 servings: meat, poultry, fish, dry beans, eggs, and nuts
2–3 servings: milk, yogurt, cheese
Use only sparingly: fats, oils, sweets

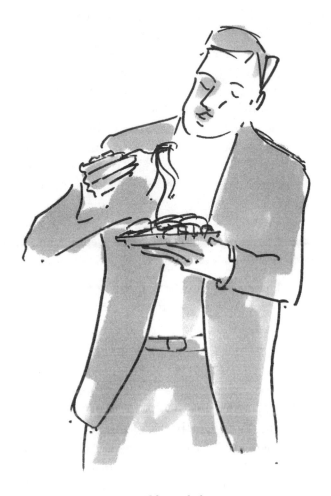

Chow, baby.

Keep in mind that a serving, in the USDA's mind, is only 3.5 ounces of meat, poultry, or fish, or half a cup of anything else. Translated, one serving of turkey is about the size of a deck of cards, cut in half.

Ornish's diet would consist of more fruits and vegetables, no meat, and much less fat. How much do you need to worry? To answer that question, consider your shape. Your *real* shape.

Recent studies have shown that if you carry a ton of weight in your gut, then you've got the typical male problem, what they call the apple shape and that you're more likely to have high cholesterol levels, stroke, heart disease, high blood pressure, and diabetes. No one is certain of the reason for this dangerous correlation, but doctors speculate that it's because the type of fat that gathers in the midsection, "brown fat," is more active than the "white fat" found in the rest of the body, perhaps enhancing the development of the most dangerous type of cholesterol.

Ornish's diet might look even more attractive if you've got a family history of heart disease, if you have a cholesterol higher than 200 mg/dl, or if you smoke, drink, and don't work out much.

Can I lose weight, keep it off, and be healthy with the right diet even if I don't exercise?
No.

The best fruits and vegetables
Incorporate broccoli and sweet potatoes into your diet and you've got an army of vitamins and minerals at the ready. Broccoli is packed with vitamins A, C, folic acid, and calcium (and gives the body more of them than spinach), is low in calories, may have anticancer properties, and is best (and most nutritious) eaten raw. Sweet potatoes, a great source of complex carbs, pack in antioxidants such as beta-carotene and vitamin C, plus several B vitamins, potassium, and iron.

Add papaya and you'll have all the vitamin C and beta-carotene you'll need in a day, plus potassium, folic acid, and fiber. Papaya was voted Most Nutritious Fruit by the Center for Science in the Public Interest, the nutrition watchdog group (and just like Mikey, they hate everything); why, the papain enzyme in the skin even aids digestion, tenderizes meat, smoothes skin, and when applied to a burn or minor wound, can actually help speed healing.

And when in doubt, remember that bright makes right. Foods rich in beta-carotene are bright yellow or orange; sweet red peppers have about twice the carotenoids of plain old green bell peppers; dark, leafy romaine lettuce four times that of iceberg; and pink grapefruit some two hundred times more than white. Carotenoids have been linked to reducing cancer.

Up your fiber intake

Double it. Most guys eat about seventeen grams a day. They should be eating thirty. Insoluble fiber, found in whole-grain products such as whole-wheat bread, may help you cut down on calories by giving you that full feeling, as well as providing bulk in the digestive tract; soluble fiber, found in fruits and veggies (*with* the skins), beans, cereals, and oats, may also help reduce cholesterol levels.

Ordering out

Order steamed dishes. Ask for dressing on the side. Avoid fried foods. Ask how a dish is prepared—grilled is good. And remember, a steak every once in a while won't kill you. Just don't make a steady diet of it.

How does a guy get fat on a no-fat diet?

By stuffing down a dozen bagels a day, along with a box of no-fat cookies and five platters of pasta. Stick to about 2,000 to 2,500 calories a day.

What about protein drinks, sports bars, supplement shakes, and all the other musclehead-magazine stuff? Is there any item from that category that does all it claims to do?

No. All those products that claim to whittle away fat and build muscle simply provide calories, extra energy to make you feel renewed after a workout. Of course, there's a lot to feeling renewed, and replenishing glycogen stores (which your body uses up during an intense workout) by filling up on a high-carb snack does help the body recover more quickly than it would on its own. But as for muscle building . . .

Muscle building depends on three things: genetics, testosterone, and resistance training. No sports bar contains those.

Vitamin supplements

They can't hurt—not unless you take them in absurdly high quantities (which are sometimes advocated on labels or ads for supplements in health-food stores, so watch for the hype). Taking the RDA, even twice that amount, is generally a safe, effective means of picking up the nutrients that your crappy diet leaves in the dust. However, if you're looking to gain all the vaunted health benefits of antioxidants (protection from cancer to heart disease to aging), then buckle up and drive on over to the produce section of your supermarket—because as studies consistently show, you're more likely to get the benefits you want from vitamins *inside foods* (which are chock-full of all kinds of nutrients and other useful stuff that may work in conjunction with the antioxidants—things that scientists still know little about) rather than inside pills.

DISEASE

What, you worry?

You are the owner of a marvelously resilient organism. It's called your body. And no matter how many bad movies you see about lab monkeys carrying creepy viruses that will turn people into human smoothies, chances are you're not going to die from some rare disease. (If you're still not ready to eat right and exercise and quit smoking, that's another story, and it's called heart-attack-waiting-to-happen). But as for germs, bacteria, tumors, and the like, there's a lot you don't need to worry about. Before we get to the things you *should* be scared of, let's review your insanity.

Are you a hypochondriac, or is it all
in your head?

Temporary blindness, blood in your urine, and/or fainting spells are all nature's way of telling you to *get to a doctor, pronto!* But what about other, less, uh, severe signs of distress? Does a pain in the gut mean you need an emergency appendectomy, or that you should find a girlfriend who cooks something other than fried pork jalapeños, then serves cake and peanuts for dessert? Herewith, a guide to symptoms, probable causes, and horrifying possibilities.

Backache

Probable causes: You're carrying around repressed rage, you're tense, your mattress is too soft, you overdid it at the gym, your chair at the office is too high (or low), or you have nonbacterial prostatitis.

Horrifying possibility: Cancer.

Belching and gas

Probable causes: Just switched to a diet high in fruits and vegetables, one too many Dr Peppers, pork 'n' beans.

Horrifying possibility: Peptic ulcer.

Chest pain

Probable causes: Heartburn, pulled muscle from bench-pressing too much.

Horrifying possibilities: Heart attack or coronary artery disease, pneumonia, hiatal hernia.

Constipation

Probable causes: Anxiety, not enough water, crash diet, travel.

Horrifying possibilities: Diverticulitis, your thyroid has conked out, colon cancer.

Dizziness

Probable cause: It's time for lunch.

Horrifying possibility: Brain tumor.

Recurrent headaches

Probable causes: You hate your job, you miss your girlfriend, you long for love and happiness and more meaning in your life. Also, your shirt collar is too tight.

Horrifying possibilities: Malignant brain tumor. Your shirt collar is too tight.

Fever

Probable cause: The flu.

Horrifying possibility: The plague.

Bloody stool

Probable causes: Hemorrhoids; it's not blood, you've been eating a lot of beets and cranberries lately.

Horrifying possibility: Cancer of the intestinal tract.

Suffering from something a little more exotic?

The National Organization for Rare Disorders (NORD) offers reports on more than one thousand unusual conditions, including information on symptoms, treatments, and organizations that can provide assistance. Call 1-800-999-6673.

The prostate primer

It's just an innocent little organ that produces secretions that become part of your ejaculate. It starts to grow at puberty, stops at twenty, then starts up again at fifty. It also accounts for more visits to the urologist than any other sexual health problem, especially for men in their twenties and thirties, not to mention the prevalence of cancer in older men.

First, the noncancerous diseases of the prostate.

Acute bacterial prostatitis is marked by abrupt onset of fever, chills, lower-back pain, frequent urination, and sometimes even urinary retention.

Chronic bacterial prostatitis is often marked by a series of urinary-tract infections, as well as stomach pain, pain in the lower back and testicles, and pain when urinating and ejaculating. Treatment for bacterial prostatitis means antibiotics, sometimes for as long as three months for the chronic form.

If you're a traveling salesman, marathon bike rider, or anyone who puts a great deal of pressure on his butt, you're a good candidate for *nonbacterial prostatitis*.

For nonbacterial prostatitis, you'll probably be told to avoid alcohol and spicy foods, to have sex as often as you'd like, and maybe even to take a nonsteroidal anti-inflammatory and/or hot baths. You might even be told to masturbate to relieve congestion.

As you get older, your prostate will probably start to grow again, usually at about age fifty. No one knows why it happens, but if that's all that happens, you have *benign prostatic hypertrophy* (BPH). Symptoms occur gradually, as the ringlike prostate slowly squeezes and distorts the urethra. Urine flow is obstructed or weak, yet you feel like you have to go often.

Half of all men over sixty have an enlarged prostate. By the time you're eighty, chances are 90 percent that the gland is big enough to make pissing problematic, if not a pain. For many men, just an enlarged gland (BPH) is more nuisance than problem and doesn't need to be treated.

Prostate cancer is another story. It can kill you.

The most basic test is the aptly named digital rectal exam (DRE), which I think you can figure out. The more sophisticated is a blood test measuring prostate-specific antigen (PSA), a substance that works in conjunction with antibodies. High PSAs are an indication of cancer. The problem is, they are also a sign of benign prostate enlargement, and the PSA cannot distinguish between the two. It also can't differentiate between a dangerous, spreading tumor and one that will stay localized and harmless.

A high PSA might lead to a biopsy or other test. Further treatment options include shrinking, irradiating or removing the gland, as well as toasting it with a heated probe inserted through the urethra, balloon dilation to widen the urinary passage, and coring it with an instrument called a resectoscope, inserted up the penis and urethra. Many physicians are now prescribing prostate-shrinking drugs, as well as other drugs that relax the muscle tissue in the prostate and urinary tract, which make emptying the bladder easier.

Treatment risks include impotence, sterility, incontinence, decreased libido, and low blood pressure. Not to mention death on the operating table. The good news is that prostate cancer, like BPH, operates on a slow growth curve. About 30 to 50 percent of prostate-cancer patients die from something else first.

Annual screening for prostate cancer should begin in your forties if you're black or you have a family history of the disease. Otherwise, you're probably safe waiting until fifty.

Whatever age you are, eat lots of grains, fruits, and vegetables. And try to avoid large amounts of fat, especially the type found in red meat. It's been linked to higher incidences of prostate cancer.

High-tech blues

Your wrists are numb. Your fingers hurt. When you go to sleep at night, tiny shocks of pain play tag up and down your arms. Welcome to the brave new world of computers, cyber-boy. With so many men behind keyboards these days, carpal tunnel syndrome (CTS) is no longer solely the affliction of meat cutters and others who perform the same motions day after day. This might bring butchers joy, but for you, it's a pain, literally.

While CTS gets most of the headlines, it's just one of many repetitive strain injuries (RSIs) often caused by overuse or improper placement of computer keyboards and laptop computers. To guard against getting an RSI, don't rest your arms while you type. You wouldn't throw a baseball with just wrist action (or at least your ball wouldn't get very far if you did); same thing with typing or moving the mouse. The small muscles and tendons in your wrist shouldn't be doing all the work. Make the bigger muscles in your hand and arm labor a little, too.

If you think you've got CTS, consult a physical therapist for exercises. Also be prepared to take long breaks from the computer.

TO SLEEP, PERCHANCE TO DREAM
ZZZZZZZZZZZZZZZZ

When was the last time you had a good night's sleep? If you can answer "last night," skip this section. If it's been a couple of weeks, help is at hand. And if you can't remember, and furthermore, you're sure that the old guy in the next apartment is beaming control rays at you through your toaster, this might be a good time to put down the book and see a doctor.

Insomnia can hurt work performance, strain your relationships ("What do you mean, 'How am I?' What the hell kind of question is that? Can't you just *leave me alone!*"), pose harm (fifty-six thousand auto accidents annually in the United States are due to driver fatigue), and, this is the real drag, make you tired all the time.

If you have transient insomnia, it's probably due to a change in schedule, a new girlfriend, jet lag, or a problem at work. Don't worry about it.

If it lasts for weeks and it's connected to a big problem at work or illness, it's short-term insomnia. Then there's the Daddy Longlegs of sleep deprivers, chronic insomnia. It can last for months, even years, and it's the one that drives people to drink and drugs.

What to do?

First off, lay off the booze and over-the-counter medications. Alcohol, while knocking you out at first, causes sleep disturbances in the middle of the night.

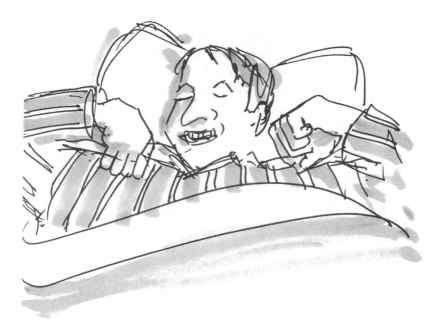

To sleep, perchance . . .

Sleeping pills, safe if used infrequently, can lead to tolerance and addiction. In fact, a lot of sleep experts say such pills are the leading cause of insomnia in the world.

Instead, stick to a set bedtime and wake-up time. Keep it even on weekends. Reserve your bedroom for sleeping and sex, only. Cut down on coffee and anything else caffeinated. (You might even need to eschew it anytime after noon.) No nicotine at least three or four hours before bed. It's a stimulant. Have a glass of milk about ninety minutes before bedtime. It contains L-tryptophan, an amino acid that will make you drowsy.

You might consider melatonin, the latest in a long line of "miracle drugs." Yes, people do report that it has helped with jet lag and insomnia. But there are no long-term studies evaluating the consequences of years of use.

Finally, if the problem is severe, there are sleep clinics in most major cities.

If you're getting seven or eight hours a night, and you skimp on a night or two, don't spend the rest of the week staring at the ceiling worrying about it. You'll live.

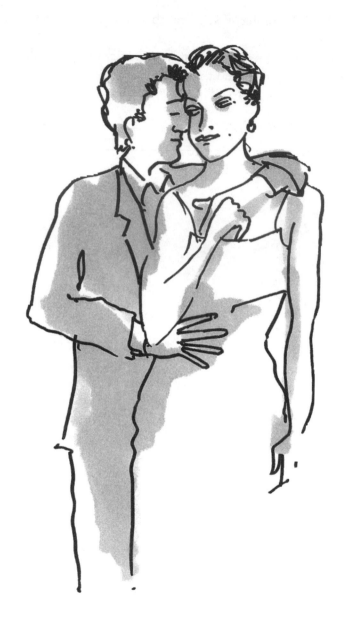

LOVING WELL

THE BOTTOM LINE

Feel her pain, touch her heart, rub her feet.

INDISPENSABLE ITEMS

Generous spirit, engaging sense of humor, charming smile, accounts at a neighborhood flower store and a romantic restaurant where the maître d' treats you like a regular, condoms.

COMMON QUESTIONS

What is this thing called love? If I can't be with the one I love, is it okay to love the one I'm with? Does sexual attraction inevitably fade? Why am I never satisfied? How do I fight fair? What's a sure sign that it's over?

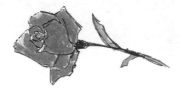

A gentleman is attuned to the needs

of others and sometimes willing to sublimate his most basic impulses and wanton desires in order to put those others at ease. This is especially true when he thinks such a head fake might get him some action. He is giving, generous, and honest, except in cases when generosity and honesty might put a serious dent in his chances of having sex with as many pretty young women as possible. A gentleman is gentle, to be sure, but he is, after all, still a man.

Sadly, some women view this essential duality of man's nature as evidence of his weaseliness. Tragically, as Christopher Lasch pointed out in his classic critique of American Society in the 1970s, *The Culture of Narcissism,* women "cultivate a protective shallowness, a cynical detachment they do not altogether feel but which soon becomes habitual and in any case embitters personal relations merely through its repeated profession."

A gentleman is saddened by this protective shallowness, this cynical detachment. A gentleman is frightened when women start glorifying and codifying such shallowness. A gentleman is truly horrified when such shallowness forms the basis of a best-seller.

Take *The Rules.* Please. In this slim and evil 1995 book, two hard-bitten New York City women offer advice to other women on how to make sure a date leads to marriage. They suggest things such as never doing more than kissing on the first date, never accepting an invitation to a weekend date if it comes after

Wednesday, never staying on the phone longer than ten minutes, and always being the one to end the telephone conversation.

A man, especially a sensitive, caring, feeling (but still manly) man, rejects such reductive and bloodless "rules" as the desperate and angry venting of two lonely and platinum-plate-hearted women. Such a man blames a fast-paced industrial society and the ever-spreading anomie that plagues our cities and robs our collective soul. (He does not blame himself or other men, though.)

Such a man knows that "rules" designed to guide women and men through the excruciatingly painful but exquisitely sweet rituals of courtship and love are hopelessly simplistic and absolutely incapable of embracing the ineffably wide range of thoughts, feelings, and actions that make us who we are.

That's why I'm calling mine "guidelines." (I'm focusing on heterosexual behavior because of sheer numbers and personal taste.)

GENERAL GUIDELINES
TO SURVIVE THE MYSTERY AND
MADNESS OF LOVE

Why do fools fall in love? Can pigs walk on two legs?
Why can't you listen?
And some other things that might come in handy.

Guideline number one—motivation matters

Here's a quiz. A man turns thirty-five, tells his girlfriend of four years that he "needs space," while instructing her to pack her things and decamp, then starts an affair with one of his employees while meeting one of his old girlfriend's old friends, who is married, for twice-a-week trysts.

Is he

a. flailing about in confusion and desperation over impending middle age and the mortality it portends, trying to silence his almost palpable terror in a series of sordid assignations with non-threatening women?

b. healthily expressing a male urge as old and as irresistible as the survival instinct itself?

c. demonstrating his caring, altruistic side, having come to the conclusion that he is not what his girlfriend needs and that in order for her to fully develop, she needs to "spread your wings, my precious sparrow, and remember, I will always be here for you"?

d. sick of her cooking?

Here's another multiple-choice test:

Are you obsessed with your girlfriend's little sister because

a. you cannot confront your fears of commitment with your girl-friend, and by focusing on her sister you can avoid examining the issues that really plague you?

b. you're healthily expressing a male urge as old and as irre-sistible as etc. . . . ?

c. you're a pig?

d. you've never been able to resist the pert way Sissy flips her hair?

If you guessed A on either test, you're wrong. If you guessed B on either or C or, for that matter, D, you're also wrong.

The fact is, when it comes to love, it's not what you do, but why you do it. Existentialists (and remember, Jean-Paul Sartre chased quite a bit of what the French call *la tail* in his day) call this the "adverbial ethic," and it can serve you well in matters of the heart. After all, doesn't it sound better to say, "But, honey, it's *why* I was flirting with that soap opera actress that matters," rather than, "Uh, me, flirting, uh, whaddya mean?"

As long as you're not breaking any laws, putting someone in a position where they're powerless to say no (someone who works for you, someone who's drunk), or behaving in a way likely to spread disease and destruction—all activities that are prima facie sleazy—the adverbial ethic applies to just about everything else. Whether you're celibate, profligate, hetero-, bi-, or homosexual, remember, it's the impulse that counts, not (necessarily) the action.

Guideline number two—it's healthy, natural,
and perfectly okay to pursue models,
actresses, homecoming queens, and other
classically beautiful women

This is so because

a. dating these women allows you to lord it over your guy friends.

b. you're an animal following urges as old and as irresistible etc. . . .

c. a classically beautiful woman with high cheekbones (as recent studies show) triggers your hardwired preference for the evolutionarily strong mate who is healthy, fertile, and unlikely to possess any genetic anomalies. As for those widely (but not too widely) spaced blue eyes and long legs, those are plugging into your unconscious (until now) taste for bilateral symmetry—which studies show predicts better health, more sexual activity, and greater likelihood (in women) of climax during intercourse.

Guideline number three—it's also perfectly
fine to pursue Hilda from accounting,
the one with the sensible shoes and
Phi Beta Kappa key ring

If you're moving on Marian the librarian, you're a smart man, because

a. competition is limited.

b. research suggests that children inherit their intelligence from their mothers, not their fathers. So if you want some thinking kids, you should be checking the symmetry of her brain hemispheres, not her extremities.

c. when she lets down her hair and flings her glasses across the room, you like it.

SOME QUESTIONS ABOUT LOVE AND LUST EVERY MAN SHOULD CONSIDER

There are no right answers. Some, though, will get you in more trouble than others.

Does sexual attraction inevitably fade?

A Lutheran minister told a couple I know to keep a jar and a bag of jelly beans next to their bed, and to put a jelly bean into the jar each time they had sex the first three years of their marriage. After three years, they were to start removing the jelly beans each time they had sex. "The jar will never be empty," the minister said. Now, in addition to being a real downer of a holy guy, Father Bummer was also operating under the quaint and delusional notion that they were marrying as virgins. But his point is clear.

Dr. Mark Schwartz, clinical director of the Masters and Johnson Institute, says sexual tension "has to be maintained. . . . It comes from two individuals continually growing and changing. It's being open to the process of change and not being threatened by your partner changing."

Layman's translation: "Yes, it does inevitably fade."

Or, as my late and thrice-married great-grandmother, Ida, used to tell me, "Kissing doesn't last. Cooking does."

Why is a man never satisfied?

First, see above.

Second, consider the words of Adam Phillips, who points out in *On Flirtation: Psychoanalytic Essays on the Uncommitted Life* (1994), "In so far as we value reliability and the relatively predictable, it is inevitable that flirtation—the (consciously or unconsciously) calculated production of uncertainty—will be experienced at best as superficial and at worst as cruel."

Third, remember that we are animals driven by urges as old and as irresistible . . .

So why get married?

You will always have a date Saturday night. Tax advantages. Because, as Frank Lloyd "the Lovemaster" Wright once said, "A man's love is no greater than he is. As he is, so will his love be." So you won't be fifty, eating pizza out of the box, and watching reruns of *thirtysomething* and wishing you had Hope, and hope. You want kids. Because W. B. Yeats said, "The supreme experience of life [is]: to share profound thoughts, and then to touch."

Because Antoine de Saint-Exupéry wrote, "To love does not mean so much to look at each other as to look together in the same direction," and what's marriage but looking in the same direction? Because, on a more practical note, research indicates that married men earn more money and report lower levels of alcohol and cigarette consumption, which probably explains why they also tend to live longer than their bachelor brothers.

> *Then why in the world should you*
> *stay hopelessly and sadly single, increasing*
> *your chances of early death and forever*
> *remaining the mysterious bachelor uncle*
> *at family gatherings, where you are*
> *looked upon with amusement by the little ones*
> *and not a small amount of pity by*
> *the grown-ups?*

Because this way you might get to have sex with young women who possess single-digit body fat, laughter like the chiming of church bells, and the overall friskiness of baby seals.

Do women, even eventually
the baby-seal types, really see the world in
terms of connection and feeling and
process and are men doomed to
misunderstand and inadvertently offend
and hurt their romantic partners because
we're (yeah, you and me) genetically
stuck in a tragically limited,
hopelessly rational, and conventional
way of dealing with life?

How should I know? I'm a rational guy and consequently don't
have the time for questions like that.

MEETING THE WOMAN OF YOUR DREAMS

Where, how, and when. If you don't know why, pretend.

You have pondered the guidelines of romance. The important
questions about life and love have been asked and answered.
Now you are ready to meet a woman. This is a laughably simple
task if you happen to be a European prince, a movie star, or a rock-
and-roll poet whose music touches the souls of all those who hear
it, especially the souls of young women with laughter like the
chiming of church bells. The rest of you will need some help.

Phrases to avoid in making your
initial approach

"You remind me of my mother."
"I haven't been with a woman since I got out."
"Sweet Jesus, I am in the mood for love."
"I have so much to give. I need someone who will take."
"You look like a tequila gal."

Behavior to avoid

Eyeballing that lasts more than a few minutes. "I like to feel pretty," a woman friend tells me. "I don't like to feel like I'm a lamb chop and he's getting ready for supper."

Psychologically sadistic behavior that I in no way endorse but that might make you feel better

Hang out at your local bookstore and strike up a conversation with a woman you see buying *The Rules*. Ask her out. Later call her Wednesday night/Thursday morning at 12:10 A.M., to invite her for a weekend date. Enjoy her silent but furious mental struggle. Say things like "Well, I'd better be . . ." and count how many milliseconds it takes for her to end the phone conversation.

What words and actions might actually work in getting a date with that sultry redhead you spot at the other end of the bar

"Hi."

"How are you?"

"Can I buy you a drink?"

Important thing to remember about these words

They might not work, too.

INTERPRETING YOUR DATE'S BEHAVIOR

She says, "You're really nice." You poor bastard.

So now you've seen the woman who you hope will turn out to be charming, kind, inventive in the kitchen, spiritually evolved, and gymnastically gifted in bed. (Also, you'd like her to be fond of children.) But you don't really know her. This is the purpose of dating. To make the most of this frightening but necessary ritual, you need to watch. You need to listen.

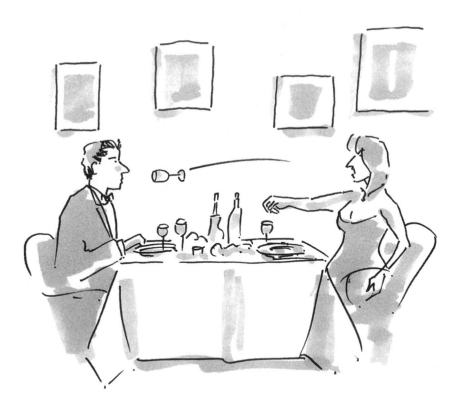

Pay attention to her subtle behavioral clues.

If she uses the words patriarchal and
oppressive in combination more than two or
three times and refers to women she
doesn't know as "my sisters"
You might want to rethink your holding-hands-on-a-moonlit-stroll-after-a-nice-bottle-of-Chianti plan.

When you pick her up at her place, and
you see stacks of Cosmopolitans
on the coffee table
You can assume that she sees men as unruly but high-earning children who will, in exchange for the promise of athletic sex with a woman who makes lots of noise, open doors, buy flowers, and propose marriage. She suspects that you might *promise* these things, in hopes of getting the athletic, noisy sex. A date with a *Cosmo* girl is an exercise in bluffing, negotiation, domination, and loss. Kind of like a spirited game of RISK, but more expensive.

When she is more than fifteen years your
junior and can't stop staring at your receding
hairline and mentions that the restaurant
you are dining at is a place she hasn't visited
"since my creepy uncle took me here"
(this happened to me)
Skip the salads and eat fast.

When she mentions her old boyfriend more
than three times, and the words animalistic,
primitive, and I was miserable, but deeply
satisfied creep into the conversation
Cut your losses.

When she stares into your eyes: that's good.
Lingering eye contact is really good. If she says,
"This is really fun," it is either very good or
the mark of someone who's dating skills are
more finely honed than yours.
Ask yourself why a woman would have finely honed dating skills.
The answer might not be pretty.

PLANNING YOUR STRATEGY

Walk like a man. Spend like a drunken sailor.
Think like a commando.

Be visionary

Assuming you like your date, you want to focus on your maturity, your sophistication, your paycheck. (Just as your brain is looking for eye-pleasing and breeding-positive symmetry, her brain, according to several women I know, is scanning for evidence of income). Feel free to express your wry wit. But in general, avoid the priest-and-the-rabbi-walking-into-the-bar joke.

Be curious

Studies prove that the more you drop the word *you* into your conversation, the more attractive you are perceived to be. There are important exceptions. In general, avoid the unvarnished "you make me hot" construction. And when she says, "What are you, a reporter/prosecutor?" that's your cue to stop grilling her. Either that, or smile playfully and say, "Does that mean you're ready to play off-the-record source/hostile witness?"

Be generous

You invited her. You pay. If she offers to split it, refuse on the first date. After that, payment should be determined by who does the inviting, who makes more money, and personal preference. If you're dating someone who makes three times as much as you and who also feels that "a man who's a real man always pays" (I dated someone like that), you might rethink things. Then again, you might be foolishly and tragically locked into the same type of outdated and repugnant sexual stereotyping that she is. I make no judgments about that.

Be cool, but not too cool

"Everybody's socially anxious on a . . . date," says Debra A. Hope, expert in social anxiety and director of the psychological consultation center at University of Nebraska, Lincoln. "It's normal. If you're not somewhat nervous, it's a little bit of a concern. Most women's reaction to a man being a little nervous is positive. Not nervous at all comes across as arrogant." ("A little nervous" does not mean you should say, "Jeez, Louise, you make me sweat a lot.")

Be a man with a plan

Don't say, "So what do you wanna do?" Have reservations.

Don't talk about your old girlfriend

Under no circumstances mention that she was "a drag in bed." This is disrespectful of women and can be intimidating.

Don't mention your mother too often

Limit your remarks to innocuous phrases like "She's really nice" and "When you're talking lasagna, you're talking mom's language." Avoid words such as *psycho* and *smothering*. Definitely do not say, "I want to forgive her, but it's hard, really, really hard."

Don't check out other women

If you must, be discreet. This means tracking with eyes only. No head movement, and definitely no slack jaws combined with exclamations like "Holy Mother of God!"

Do not mention Soldier of Fortune *magazine*
It's worse than *Cosmo*. Much worse.

Do not say, at the end of the evening,
"I dropped forty bucks and I don't even
get a kiss?"
Never admit defeat.

THE BLIND DATE

Remember, lunch only takes an hour.

L et's say the model you ran into at the dry cleaners didn't melt
when you said hello to her. Let's assume, in fact, that you're
neither royalty, a rock star, a male model, or surrounded by familiar
and appealing women who are constantly asking you out. Let's say
you're about to spend a few hours with someone you've never laid
eyes on. Let's not say you're a chump, though we are thinking
exactly that.

If you are a guy going on a blind date, you possess a desperate
and fevered imagination. You have chosen to ignore the wealth of
statistical data (compiled by my friends and me) that demonstrates
conclusively that blind dates lead most often to fear and loathing,
occasionally to a semipleasant evening, and almost never to any
kind of happy connection. Then again, there is the "desperate"
angle at work. So . . .

Learn the language
To the untrained ear "I think she's attractive" is a harmless, even
pleasant sentiment. To the steel-trap brain of the single guy, a
wondrous organ that can perform precise and instantaneous gram-
matical deconstruction, it is a death knell, and it's tolling for thee,

big guy. Why did your matchmaking friend say "I think"? And why choose "attractive" over "pretty"? The answer is plain.

Other phrases that should prompt an "Uh, maybe I should spend more time alone, working on *me*" response:

"She's got beautiful skin." "She's got really nice eyes." (In fact, the word *nice* should set off alarm bells whenever you hear it.) "I think she's really fun." Words that would be laughable if they weren't so tragic, and that I promise I've heard before: "Great personality," "She's a big girl," and "She kind of hates men, but . . ."

Consider the source

Is the person doing the fixing up a friend of yours or a friend of hers? More to the point, does he/she owe you a favor? If not, guess what? If you go on this date, you're the favor.

Be flexible

Once I was fixed up with the granddaughter of a famous advice columnist. I figured she would be either horribly conventional or perpetually angry and maladjusted. I came prepared for either. When I saw the scowling brunette in the motorcycle jacket slouching at the jukebox, sucking on a Camel and nursing a manhattan, I removed my blue blazer to reveal a torn black T-shirt, then started complaining, in world-weary tones, about the yuppies and other hopelessly bourgeois elements ruining the neighborhood. Bingo.

Be decent

There's nothing wrong with having sex on the first date. There is something wrong with saying "I love you," and then never calling again.

MAKING THE FIRST MOVE

So what if it's risky? It's your only choice.

The man who is sensitive to environmental stimuli and attuned to subtle behavioral cues will often decide early on in the dating process that sex would be a good idea. After the one-eighth of a second that it usually takes a man to reach such a decision, however, he is faced with a bewildering array of options and tactics involving this most sacred act.

First of all, in most cases, you, the sensitive and attuned fellow, must make the first move. Why? Because, in the words of Aaron Kipnis, director of the Gender Relations Institute in Santa Barbara, California, "Men are told, 'Be a football hero, play hard, risk death and pain, suppress all your feelings and fears. You're responsible for initiating sexual contact, and if you don't, you're a wimp, but if you do it wrong, you're a jerk.'"

With those encouraging words in your ears (why are guys who head Gender Relations Institutes never much fun?), this is what you need to know about right moves and wrong moves.

Kiss her

Cradle her face in your hands. Women like that. Don't ask me why.

Tell her you haven't felt this way in a long time as you take her in your arms

By "long time," don't mean last weekend, when you were making out with your secretary.

Be honest and forthright

But don't mention that the reason the service at the restaurant was so slow is because you slept with your waitress last week and never called her.

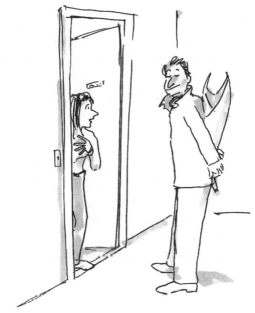

Act sweet, and she might actually think you are.

Be sincere
Or at least fake it well.

Don't put your tongue in her ear

Don't grope

Don't ask if you can kiss her
It looks sweet in coming-of-age movies. But you're not moving in on a fifteen-year-old. Are you? *Are* you?

Do nothing
A colleague who claims that every woman he wants ends up throwing herself at him says his secret is utter inaction, combined with deep gazing into the woman's eyes and expressing interest in her life. The psychodynamics behind this are twofold, women tell me.

First, the woman feels like this guy likes them for who they are and what they say, not just how they look, so they like him back, in a comfortable and easy way. Second, after a while they become worried about their attractiveness because he isn't making a move, so they make one. The downside is, it takes time.

> *Proclaim on your first date that "sex*
> *before you really get to know someone can*
> *really harm a relationship; I believe in a*
> *more organic process, a gentle*
> *unfolding of feeling"*

This operates much like doing nothing, only in a more overtly and aggressively deceptive way. The downside is that many women will see right through you.

KISSING

Saying volumes without words.

Y ou've made the move. It's worked. Resist the temptation to fall to your knees and thank the God of your religion. Instead, think about kissing for a moment.

"We most often touch a lover's genitals before we actually see them," writes Diane Ackerman in *A Natural History of the Senses*. ". . . But kissing can happen right away. . . . There are wild, hungry kisses or there are rollicking kisses, and there are kisses fluttery and soft as the feathers of cockatoos."

There are also lame, loutish, and otherwise loserlike kisses. You want to keep women away? Then ram your tongue down their throats. Or slobber on their faces. Or do a Hollywood-in-the-fifties, lockjawed, teeth-grinding smooch.

If, on the other hand, you'd be delighted if you could touch a woman's heart by first touching mouths, then follow this advice:

Be gentle
Start slow. At first, a little nibbling at the most.

Be responsive
Wait for her tongue. When it comes into your mouth, you feel like Sally Field (she likes me, she really likes me). Instead of jumping up and down, start reciprocating. Remember, gentle. Until she gets rough.

Be willing to learn
Dr. Mark Schwartz of the Masters and Johnson Institute recommends Al Pacino in *Sea of Love* as a good role model. Also, check out Warren Beatty in *Shampoo*.

Control yourself, you animal
You are not Hannibal Lecter. "When I'm having sex with guys," a woman I know tells me, "when we're actually doing it, if we're kissing, it always turns into this nondescript face smashing, 'cause they're so involved with what's going on down there. I wish guys would concentrate on the kiss a little, even during those moments of truth for them. Otherwise, just move your damn mouth away."

And don't forget the cradling-her-face-in-your-hands trick

Fun anthropological kissing perspective
"The lips remind us of the labia, because they flush red and swell when they're aroused, which is the conscious or subconscious reason women have always made them look even redder with lipstick. . . . So, anthropologically at least, a kiss on the mouth, especially with all the plunging of tongues and the exchanging of saliva, is another form of intercourse, and it's not surprising

that it should make the mind and body surge with gorgeous sensations."
—*A Natural History of the Senses*

Fun psychological interpretation of kissing

"Kissing is the sign of taming, of controlling the potential—at least in fantasy—to bite up and ingest the other person."
—*On Kissing, Tickling and Being Bored* by psychoanalyst Adam Phillips

Fun kissing question

"Is kissing a publicly permissible indulgence in foreplay, an analogy to intercourse? Is kissing a way to connect and communicate or a way to silence rational thought's annoying flow of words?"
—*A Natural History of the Senses*

Fun answer

Uh, yep.

GOOD SEX

Oh, so this is why fools fall in love.
Congratulations. The kiss worked. Now you're in the sack.

Pay attention

If she is staring at the ceiling, glassy-eyed, and/or muttering repeatedly, "I'm sorry, Jesus, I'm sorry," or even worse, "Why me, why me?" you might ask her if anything's wrong. If, on a happier note, she is saying "oooh" often and grabbing you with vigor, repeat whatever you are doing.

Be sweet

"You are so beautiful" sounds ludicrously insincere, I know, but that's because you're a guy. If you say it without laughing, she'll probably buy it. Attach her name to the end of the sentence, and you're talking fat city.

Be giving

"Get her off first," says a friend who is known in publishing circles as "The Hound," "then you'll get yours, in spades."

Be reassured that sex will get better

You'll grow to like each other more, feel more comfortable with each other, learn each other's favorite things. So relax. This is not a competition.

Be observant, but not too observant, considerate, but not too considerate

Don't be too caring a lover, says no less an authority than Virginia Johnson, of Masters and Johnson, because "the minute you start watching yourself, you cease to live. Your behavior ceases to be an honest expression of what's going on inside you."

A good solution to the Zen riddle posed by Johnson on how to synthesize the most selfish of impulses with the most heartfelt and at the same time strategic aim to please

Oral sex.

Something to remember about sex

Remember that to some people, physical union is a near-religious experience, to be practiced only when accompanied by love and deep feeling and/or alone. To others, it's as serious as jogging. It's best when both partners see it the same way.

And speaking of the clitoris

Sigmund Freud argued that a woman who comes when her clitoris is stimulated is experiencing an "immature" orgasm. Nearly a century later, it turns out, penis envy isn't the only thing that the wacky stogiemeister was wrong about. Stimulating that little pink nub of tissue (about the size of a pencil eraser, hard to find, so ask) is the surest way to give a woman an orgasm. In fact, a lot of women demand it. As Freud himself might have said, "Oy."

BAD SEX

At least make sure it's not all your fault.

Don't skip foreplay
Quickies are okay, once in a while. As a steady practice, they'll get you a quick boot.

Don't be mechanical
Sex is not like making your favorite move to the hoop (and I hope you don't say, "He shoots, he scores," when you're with her). A well-orchestrated series of head fakes and hand movements might work the first time. After a few times, they seem like a well-orchestrated series of head fakes and hand movements.

Don't coach
But do tell her what you like. There is a difference.

Don't play rough
Unless she wants you to play rough.

Don't talk dirty
Unless you have strong indications, or a strong gut feeling, that she would like it. According to "Jake" in *Glamour* (April 1996), "Talking dirty can be seductive if there is emotional buildup and sexual anticipation." Do you want to depend on a guy named Jake from *Glamour*?

Don't ask for a blow job
Do not guide her head in that direction. And remember, says a hard-driving female public relations executive I have futilely asked out many, many times, "the ponytail is not a stick shift."

Don't have sex on the first date
Unless she really looks hot.

Don't call her by someone else's name
Unless it's "honey" or "sweetie."

Don't ask her if she enjoyed herself
It's pathetic.

***Don't proclaim, "Boy, I haven't done that
in a while," then stretch and go check
out the fridge***
(A woman said and did that to me once.)

***Don't say, twenty minutes after blastoff,
"Well, I'd better get going now," and leave***
That triggers women's ancient abandonment issues old as the
African veld from whence we all sprang. You will be sorry.

DISEASE AND CONDOMS

Be afraid. But don't be ridiculous.

If you have unprotected sex, you probably won't get the AIDS
virus. In fact, if you have regular old condomless vaginal intercourse (time to get clinical here) a single time with a woman who
doesn't use intravenous drugs, your chances of getting the HIV
infection are about one in 5 million (comparably speaking, a
woman's chances are greater). The chances of catching the virus
from one exposure to an infected partner are one in five hundred.
The risks rise when you move to New York City from Fargo, North
Dakota, because the virus is more prevalent and concentrated in
certain areas than others, but that's not the important point. The
good news is, if you're a heterosexual sleeping with nondrug-using
women, you probably won't get HIV.

The bad news is, if you don't use a condom, you likely will get something else—something like venereal warts, chlamydia, genital herpes, gonorrhea, hepatitis—well, the list goes on and it's not a pretty one. How prevalent are these afflictions? Estimates on herpes range that from one in six to one in three adults in the general population carry it.

These diseases can cause sterility, arthritis, and blindness, not to mention a lot of discomfort. Oftentimes, the woman you're sleeping with will show no symptoms or be unaware of her symptoms (the same applies to you). The lesson is: Don't leave home without your rubbers. Oh, yeah, and there's the matter of babies, too.

Now that you know why to wear a condom,
here are a few other things to think about

Lambskin condoms are not proven to prevent the transmission of viruses. Stick with latex.

If you have a condom without a reservoir tip, leave one-half inch of space.

Toss them if the expiration date is past or if the manufacture date is more than four years ago. (You been living in a monastery or something?)

Wallets and glove compartments are handy, but they're too hot for storage.

Discussing disease

You're embarrassed? You don't want to offend her? You don't know her that well? You're afraid she'll reject you when you tell her you have something? These all are real concerns. They're also really stupid excuses for putting you and/or your partner at risk of catching something that might be chronic, painful, sterility producing, sometimes incurable and/or terminal.

Broach the subject thusly: "This feels serious. I want us to be monogamous. And I want us to feel safe with each other. I think

we should talk about our sexual history." If it's just a fling, leave out
the mushy stuff and get straight to the point.

MOVING TO SOMETHING A LITTLE MORE SERIOUS

You like her. You really, really like her.

In a perfect world, you and your honey aren't sleeping together
until you feel emotionally secure with each other, until you have
felt a deepening and enriching respect for each other's values, and
until you share a vision of a future together. At least in a perfect
world as envisioned by the grandparents of the woman you're having sex with, Billy Graham, and Mu'ammar Gadhafi. But the truth
is, sometimes you have sex with someone before you're sure you
want a future with them. That's fine. But what happens when
you do want to progress to the next level? There are a few things
you can do. Here are three.

Cook for her

Stay away from chili, spaghetti, and scrambled eggs. If she's older
than seventeen (and if she's not, you might want to check out your
state's statutory rape laws), other guys have already prepared these
hearty, nutritious, and lame-ass concoctions. Plus they're sloppy
and the chili might produce unfortunate digestive consequences.

No, what you want is something elegant, something light,
something that says, "I care enough about you to spend some time
in the kitchen. Food to me is about more than eating, it is about
sensuality and sharing. It is about the heart as well as the stomach.
It is about love."

So nix on the pizza and Chinese.

Here's what you do. Get some nice silverware. Get some nice
plates. Get some glasses that don't have pictures of Fred and
Barney on them. Buy a candle.

Now call Mom and ask her for help. She will be delighted. She wants it to work.

Don't forget the wine. Or dessert.

And if you're serious about learning to cook (it can save you money as well as making friends and influencing people), buy *The Joy of Cooking*. It's still a classic. Or, if your time is more limited, get Pierre Franey's *The Sixty-Minute Gourmet*.

Give her a massage

With Swedish massage, you employ long strokes away from the heart toward the extremities. Shiatsu is a Japanese brand of massage in which intense pressure is applied to specific points on the body to release tension. Lomilomi is an ancient Hawaiian massage based on the long and sweeping movements of the hula dance.

And all that knowledge and a buck will get you a cup of coffee. No, the only thing you need to know about massage, romancewise, is this:

Long and hard is better than short and wimpy. If you promise a massage, she wants a rubdown, pal, not a few halfhearted squeezes and caresses from someone acting as if he has carpal tunnel syndrome. Ten-minute minimum. Beyond twenty, you're creating a monster.

Take her backpacking

There is nothing so romantic as feeling the caress of alpine breezes on your face as you look up at a blanket of stars and listen to the gentle burble of a stream near your campsite. And there is nothing so maddening as tramping through the great outdoors with a kvetch. If you're taking her hiking, you need to take the responsibility for making sure she's having a great time.

(This advice is based on age-old sexual stereotypes and the worst kind of sweeping generalizations about men, women, and the great outdoors, and it comes with apologies to my college girlfriend, who had to pull me three miles through thigh-deep snow

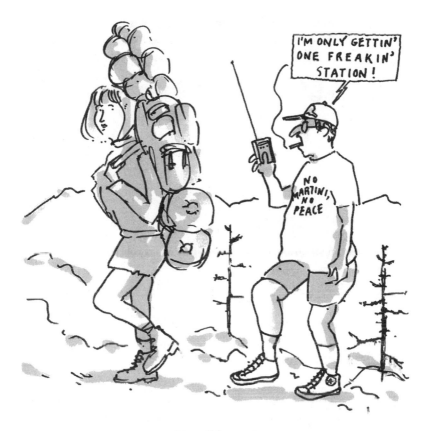

Ah, wilderness!

and a raging blizzard because I had blisters and had drunk half a
bottle of brandy "to keep warm" before we set off.)

So help her buy good hiking boots and a backpack. And make
sure she walks at least a few miles a day for a few weeks before you
hit the road.

Have a plan. It will reassure her to know you're headed to an ice
blue mountain lake nestled at the bottom of a crystal clear water-
fall. (But make sure that it's not more than six or eight miles in;
this is her first trip.)

Bring treats. Chocolate is one of the best.

Stop and smell the wildflowers. This is not a race.

Talk. She hasn't said anything for fifty-six hours? Perhaps she's been struck silent by the majesty of the meadows and the infinite beauty of the natural universe. Or maybe she hates the freeze-dried gruel you've been serving the past three days. Ask her if anything's wrong.

Don't tell her ghost stories at night, especially the couple-runs-out-of-gas-and-serial-ax-murderer-is-on-the-loose one.

Don't say, "You don't mind if I fart in the tent, do you?"

COMMITMENT

Fleeing it, seeking it, living with it.

She has eaten your food, felt your massage, slept in your tent. Now you are in big trouble. Now she wants commitment. And you might not. Why are you behaving like such an animal? Because you *are* an animal (not swine, though, despite what your girlfriend might say), and as such, you are a slave to your most primitive drives. For our cave-dwelling forefathers, the more women they could impregnate, the greater the chances their DNA would march on into the future. Behaviorally, the most successful cave guy was not the one sitting home with the wife, playing rocks. No, he was the Neanderthal out chasing other cavewomen.

The most successful cavewomen, though, was the one who could raise the most children, and that meant keeping cave guy around to protect and support the mewling brood.

Now, flash forward a few million years. You feel an urge to have sex with women you don't know. Your girlfriend/wife wants you to stay home or to accompany her and Junior to the corner ice-cream store. Both of you are expressing age-old drives. This anthropological wisdom will help you understand why men and women approach commitment differently. It will not be a good idea to mention it to most women.

To get you to increase your commitment
level, she might

Play hard to get.

Cook well.

Laugh at your jokes.

Mention that she's met a French documentary filmmaker and that "he's interesting, in a European kind of way."

Get pregnant.

Help you.

Inspire you.

Understand you.

Love you.

Make you love her.

Or she might say some things to up
the ante, things like

"Wouldn't it be fun to go somewhere together over the weekend?"

"How do you really feel about me?"

"I want you to meet my parents."

"Wouldn't it make sense to cut our rental costs in half?"

"Let's get a dog."

"I'm pregnant."

"Let's spend Thanksgiving together."

"Do you ever think about the difference in our religions?"

"What do you think our children would look like?"

Or, against the laws of nature, but in an
all-too-common scenario in these modern
times, you might decide you want to
increase the chances that she'll commit
to you. In that case, you can

Love her.

Tell her you love her.

Impregnate her. ("At least ten times as effective as flowers," according to a colleague who recently became a husband and father.)

MEETING HER PARENTS

They're older than you. They're smarter than you.
You're in big trouble.

Rule number one: Don't do it

Even if you're "serious" about the woman you're dating, and that means, at the very least, that you can say the word *girlfriend* without feeling a sharp pain in your stomach. Even if you're mutually, firmly, and definitely "not serious" about each other and your presence is only as a friend. Even if she tells you, "It's no big deal." Come to think of it, *especially* if she tells you it's no big deal.

Now that you've ignored rule number one

Find out her father's occupation and what sports teams he likes. If he's a St. Louis Cardinals fan, and between forty and sixty, express admiration for Bob Gibson. On second reference, call him (Gibson) Hoot. Be cognizant of the team's standing and have a few opinions about their current slump. (Hint: Railing against the high salaries of "today's ballplayers" usually strikes a responsive chord.)

What you're shooting for with Mom is earnest, but not slippery. Beaver Cleaver is okay. Eddie Haskell is not. "Now I see where Mary got her looks, Mrs. D." might work. "Boy oh boy, Mrs. D., I thought you were Mary's sister" is nauseating.

Also, eat whatever she gives you. Ask for seconds.

When you look at their daughter, try to appear dreamy

But do not ever refer to her as "my little filly."

Beware of parental behavior that includes

The father yelling at, ignoring, or generally treating the mother poorly. This is bad.

The mother doing that to Dad. This is really bad.

Mom flirting with you. This is disturbing.

Dad kissing your girlfriend. On the lips. For a long time. This is really disturbing.

Dad kissing you. On the lips, etc. Really, really disturbing.

Either or both crying a lot and calling you "Son."

And beware of parental language that includes

Frequent use of the phrase "your people."

Repeated queries about your age.

Relentless questions about "your intentions."

THE BOYFRIEND/GIRLFRIEND PARADIGM

One might be the loneliest number, but two comes with its share of headaches.

Now that you're part of a couple, there are certain things you can and cannot do. You cannot have sex with whomever you want. This prohibition violates your age-old genetic imperatives and causes a great deal of psychic pain, and maybe you should have thought about it a little harder before you agreed to meet her parents, you dope. I warned you.

But what's past is past. So what if you can't watch the Classic Sports Channel on Saturday night while you eat pizza with the guys, then go to a topless club afterward where you can chat with Shanna, your favorite dancer, who seems to radiate a fundamental decency that you alone can see and who you think would really like you if only you two could spend some time together? You're a boyfriend now. You get to bask in the glow emanating from the love you share with your sweetheart. You get to say you have a sweetheart. You must be in, or at least near, love, otherwise this deal would not sound so great to you.

If you want to keep your sweetheart, you must master some practices and procedures. They include:

Valentine's Day and her birthday

Surprises are key. Even if you're just taking her out to dinner and a show, the fact that she doesn't know *which* restaurant and *what* show will whet her curiosity. But give her a hint of what to wear. Even though you feel at home anywhere in your khakis and Hawaiian shirt with the pictures of battling swordfish wearing sunglasses, women hate feeling overdressed, underdressed, or generally unprepared. (And put on a coat and tie, for God's sake.) Send the flowers to her work, not home. She'll get fussed over and her friends and coworkers will think you're a prince.

When choosing a gift, think personal and specific. You met in an acting class when she played Stella to your Stanley Kowalski? Buy her a first edition of A *Streetcar Named Desire*, with a mushy note. Also give her some colored crepe that you can hang over a bare lightbulb later.

You both love the Yankees? Move heaven and earth to get an eight-by-ten of Wade Boggs, with a personal inscription. She misses her folks in Kentucky? Get her salt and pepper shakers in the shape of the Bluegrass State and bake her the cookies she loves most, from a recipe you get from her mother. (You are scoring off the chart on this one. If and when you break up, it will not be quick and painless.)

These personalized, specific, heartrendingly intimate and loving gifts work wonders. They do not, however, get you off the hook in the coming-up-with-some-things-that-cost-cash category.

Those demand special attention.

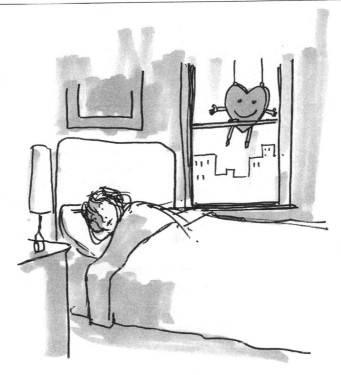

Surprises are key.

Lingerie

Never ask a woman what size lingerie she wears. Instead, check out her underwear for size *and* brand. This is not to duplicate the brand (she wants something new, chucklehead, and not something she would buy for herself), but to share that information with the salesperson.

Remember, you're buying this for her, not your fantasy woman. Thongs and rough lace and slimy synthetics and stays like phone cable won't be pleasurable for long.

Flowers

When you say it with red roses, what you're saying is "I am an unimaginative and borderline cheesy clown." It says, "I've done this before." On the other end of the spectrum is the desperately-seeking-boyish-charm approach. But only the most naive woman will fall for the bunch of daisies picked from the traffic median on your way over, or, just a step up, the tulips from the corner green-grocer. (Naive *does* have its own allure, though.)

Find out what she likes. And get some special touches put on there. Tie a nosegay of wildflowers with straw. Have the florist put in some pussy willows with the violets. And make sure you cover the details. If the flowers will need a vase and you're sending them to her office, include a vase in the order.

Candy
Chocolate.

Jewelry
Simple and elegant is better than gaudy. Gold versus silver depends on the woman. A little something is better than nothing. A ring says a lot. Make sure you mean it.

Books
Happy and reasonably sane women seem to go for Paul Auster, Laurie Colwin, and Jane Austen.

If you're dating someone with a history of psychiatric illness or what she calls "issues" and other people refer to as "an edgy nature," try *Letters to a Young Poet* by Rainer Maria Rilke, *Bastard out of Carolina* by Dorothy Allison, or anything by Sylvia Plath.

WHEN THE HONEYMOON'S OVER

People warned you there would be problems. They were right.

Fighting Fair
Be direct, be clear, be nice. Know the things that will cause irreparable harm and avoid bringing them up at all costs. If you're afraid to admit that you're hurt or feel unloved or you need her,

that means you *should* admit it. The way she hums when she pours coffee isn't *really* what's bugging you.

When she's got a problem

When she tells you her problems and cries, she doesn't necessarily want advice. She wants you to understand, to commiserate, sometimes to practice a quirky technique women refer to as "listening." This means that while your pal Andy's tale of a psychopathic boss or a cheating girlfriend can always be taken care of with a simple "Screw the bastard" or "Dump the bitch," when your sweetheart is troubled, it's a little more complicated.

How to listen

Do not speak. This is a critical first step.

Do not watch television while she speaks, even if it is the seventh game of the World Series, even if it is the season premiere of *Silk Stalkings*. (College basketball's Final Four is another matter.)

Do not ask if she minds if you turn the TV on while she speaks. Do not bleat, "Even if I turn the sound off?" This will make you heartless and pathetic. That's a combination you want to avoid.

Do not suggest that anything is her fault.

Do not offer a plan of attack.

Do not say "Is that it?" or "Is that all?" or "Can I watch the game now?"

Do hold her hand.

Do adopt an expression that shows concern and love. Maybe this is narrowed eyes. Or a slightly wrinkled forehead. Practice in front of the mirror.

If you actually *are* listening, you will score huge points later on if you can demonstrate your attentiveness. She was complaining about her older sister's incessant bossiness? When you both see someone acting dictatorially, say, "Boy, she's worse than your older sister." She mentions that violets make her weep with joy? Buy her violets.

When you do something selfish, duplicitous, and/or hurtful and you get caught

It's because you're a screwup.

When she does something selfish, duplicitous, and/or hurtful and she gets caught

It's because she was trapped in the grip of a force much larger than any force that a single human being could resist, a force so large that to try to understand it would be futile and horribly unfair to her. So the fact that you see that force as something along the lines of "you were just attracted to that asshole with the goatee and wanted to flirt" or "you really wanted to spend $700 from our joint checking account on a pair of shoes 'cause you liked them" reveals nothing so much as evidence of your testosterone-driven and pathetically narrow-minded view of the world and her. So don't even bring it up.

"I understand" is your safest bet.

When she says "I love you"

A reply is in order.

When she says, "Do you love me?"

An enthusiastic reply is in order.

Excuses for your loutish behavior that probably won't work but might be worth a try anyway

"I was following urges and instincts as old and as irresistible as, etc."

"I was frightened by the depth of my love for you. That fear made me try to sabotage our relationship. Can you forgive me?"

"Oh, yeah, well, what about the time you were flirting with that asshole with the goatee?"

"I didn't think you would care. It's not like you've shown me much feeling lately."

"I've never been involved in something so intense. I think it scared me and this was my way of trying to deal with that fear. Will you forgive me?"

"It was stupid. Can you forgive me?"

"I was running from myself."

"She means nothing."

"You're upset. Does this mean you love me?"

"I was wrong. You were right. I'll never do it again."

"I'm sorry" is the last resort. But remember, it's like penicillin. Use a minimal dose. You don't want to create an apology-resistant girlfriend/wife.

> *Newspaper column excerpt to read—and*
> *reread—to yourself the next time you think*
> *maybe it would be best to admit to your*
> *wife the time you cheated on her, because*
> *women are understanding and your wife*
> *would forgive you*

". . . I secretly wish that once, poor Lee, poor Hillary, or poor Eileen would step up to the bouquet of microphones and let loose: 'I'd like to tie that pathetic loser to a stake in the boiling sun and pour honey on his face and let red ants eat his eyes out.'

"Standing by your man is the oldest way of sacrificing your self-esteem. Instead of treating a reckless, feckless mate like a dip in the partnership's fortunes, why not send the bum packing. . . ?"

—Maureen Dowd, writing in the *New York Times*, a few days after reports that political consultant Dick Morris had behaved like a dick

BREAKING UP

The fact is, it doesn't have to be hard to do.

A re you the kind of guy who is confronting this problem often? Are you one of the men described by Schwartz of Masters and Johnson, guys "trained in the concept of conquest, who at work are attempting to fight a war, and if there isn't a challenge, they are going to create one . . . [who] will come in and conquer and destroy and improve and increase and surmount . . . [who] gets into relationships and treats the other person the same way he treats [work goals], and he's pretty unhappy."

Are you overly fond of your freedom? Do you call it "my freedom"? Do you insist that your golf buddies refer to you as "lone wolf"? Do you refer to your friends' wives as "the ol' ball and chain"? Like to listen to "Desperado" and "Don't Fence Me In" while you envision Friday night with Shanna? Do you actually use the phrase "pussy whipped"?

Or are you just drawn to single-digit body fat and laughter like the chiming of church bells?

Yes answers mean you have probably been through this breaking up thing before.

Here are some ways to make it easier.

Inoculate her

When you meet someone you like, make sure to mention that you and your longtime sweetheart have recently split up. Imply that you are bravely getting over it, but that you're in pain. That way, when you want out, you merely say, "I thought I was over her but I'm not. I'm sorry. I never wanted to hurt you."

This is appalling. It is also effective.

Another preemptive approach involves naked but tactical honesty. Say, "I don't have a very good track record with relationships, and while I want this to work, I want to be honest with you from the beginning." This releases you from all claims of liability, and as

a bonus, it can act like catnip to women who are afraid of commitment themselves, and/or those who are just busting for a challenge.

The downside to this approach is that women who *do* want
a healthy, committed relationship won't go out with you, and
then you'll be doomed to dating women who only want weird,
commitment-phobic guys. At some point, you'll have to face the
fact that you are one of these guys.

Finally, use the old "I'm starting on a big project/novel/docu-
mentary film/training regimen for the iron-man triathlon" line. If
you don't want to spend time with her after a date or two, well,
work/art/the thrill of competition is calling. If you do want to see
her more, you're not only taking her to dinner, *you're sacrificing
time spent on that which is precious to you.*

Make it her fault

Cheat on her. Be unavailable. Nod and say "Mmm-hmmm" a lot,
no matter what she is talking about. Show no interest in her crisis
at work, the invitation she received to show her film at Cannes,
the illness of her family member. When she asks if anything is
wrong, become indignant and accusatory. Say, "Why is it never
enough for you? Why can't you accept me for who I am?" Wait
until she ends things.

No man should sink this low. Many men do.

Do the right thing

If you're not a lone wolf, not terrified of marriage, not otherwise
driven by your most twisted and unconscious impulses, you might
need to break things off with someone for other, more healthy reasons. Maybe you've fallen in love with someone else, and it's not
Shanna. Maybe you've realized you'll never fall in love with her.
Maybe you caught her having sex with your best friend. In these
cases, you want to strike like the Israeli air force, or at least like it
used to. Fast, clean, surgically precise.

Be honest. Be direct. Do not whine about your pain. By no

means call her afterward "just to talk," no matter how much you miss her. That's unfair. Only call her back if you really want to make it work. Really wanting to make it work does not mean "I need sex."

Coldhearted, sleazy, and logistical considerations about breaking up

The phone is easier. It's also cowardly. Be a man.

A public place might be safer. It also is cowardly and might turn very, very ugly.

End things before your birthday and you lose out on things.

End things before *her* birthday and you'll see a net gain in your checking account.

Christmas, Valentine's Day, etc., are a wash, but when you factor in guilt and other corrosive emotions, it's probably best to get it over with.

And, speaking of what's good for the gander, phrases she says that mean you're about to get dumped

"I've been thinking . . ."

"You're really nice."

"It's not you . . ."

"Remember when I said I was going away for the weekend?"

"Remember that guy with the goatee?"

THE REAL THING?

Ain't love grand?

You've screwed up her birthday. You've gotten in fights. Maybe you've even broken up and gotten back together. You want to stay together. Why?

Because you feel a swelling in your chest when you say her name. Because you think about her often. Because some of the things about her really irritate you, and you still love her. Because you feel like you are yourself with her. Because she makes you feel brave.

Because sex is great. Because you can disagree or even fight and still love each other. Because you feel safe with her. Because you have similar values, and at least one of you laughs at the other's jokes.

Because she doesn't think what you do for a living is hopelessly stupid or corrupt, and you think her job is pretty cool, too. You want her to meet your friends. You want her to meet your parents. You want to meet her friends and family. When horrible things happen, she's there for you, and you're there for her.

Because you can envision a future together. The notion of a future apart makes you sad.

So don't screw it up.

Proposing

You could make sure the waiter brings the champagne glasses at exactly the point when the band at the Rainbow Room launches into a big-band version of the theme from *Gone With the Wind* and the helicopters you've hired buzz the windows when she takes her first sip and sees that monstrous rock at the bottom of her glass.

The downside there is, it's cash intensive. Also, if she says no, your humiliation is public.

Or, you could express white-hot love and lifelong devotion by mumbling barely articulate sentence fragments along the lines of "Uh, I was thinking, maybe you and me should spend some time together, like, uh, a lot of time, like maybe forever." If you're over twenty-three and/or don't have a goatee, forget it.

In either case, tailor the question to the respondent. She goes for pearls and wears Chanel? Down on your knees, boy.

Engagement rings

I dated a woman who one day announced that she considered marriage "a form of economic slavery." Part of me still wishes we had become husband and wife, if for no other reason than that we both saw the engagement ring as a ridiculously old-fashioned, absurdly sexist symbol of the most rigidly defined and horribly limiting kind of societal roles men and women are forced to play. Plus, I could have saved a lot of dough. Having said that, most women seem to want the damn thing.

Conventional wisdom says you should spend about two months' salary. Conventional wisdom also says you should pay attention to the "four C's"—cut, color, clarity, and carat weight. Conventional wisdom, I suspect, is written by the officers of Tiffany's and the De Beers diamond company. Make sure you spend wisely, and be sure to get papers verifying the quality of the gem and a written estimate of its value. And get the ring insured.

While diamonds are classic, sapphires and other more exotic stones are perfectly acceptable these days, especially if she thinks you had to hock something precious to afford it.

Getting the ring back

Regarding the dissolution of romance and the issue of getting the ring back, Harrier Lerner, author of *Dance of Anger* and *Life Preservers* as well as an ongoing advice column, says, "Timing and tact, and warmth, are what make honesty most possible." So if she (your fiancée, not Harriet) breaks things off, or you catch her cheating on you, tell her, with as much timing, tact, and warmth as possible, "Gimme my goddamn ring back."

THE LONG HAUL
Making love last.

In the short term, it's easy. You're charming, she's charming. You're charming together. Sex is great. Then you're busy. She's demanding. She's busy. You're cranky. You both want space. What's the secret?

Rilke wrote that

Love consists in this,
that two solitudes
protect and touch and greet each other.

So respect her dreams, make room for her hopes, ease her fears. Regard your marriage as a living, breathing entity, as precious and as fragile as a newborn baby, as wondrous as life itself. Make room for her quirks and embrace the ways in which she is different from you. Be open to the mystery of love.

In other words, get separate bathrooms.

Look, supple limbs and skin like butterscotch are nice, but to perpetually possess beauty, a man dooms himself to a sad string of shallow, transient encounters that lead to nothing but more shallow, transient encounters. Okay, so maybe that doesn't sound so bad, but it's expensive, and didn't I already warn you about how much engagement rings cost?

Besides, don't forget the health benefits that come with a lifelong companion (your health benefits, anyway; research shows that women don't benefit nearly as much from matrimony, but an institution—even a societally blessed one—can't be expected to help everyone, right?). So let's assume you want your marriage to work. That doesn't mean you can't miss those golden, beery weekends with the boys. It does mean you shouldn't proclaim—after she cooks you dinner and washes your softball uniform, and after you scratch your belly and belch—"God *damn*, I miss those golden, beery weekends with the boys."

No, the most effective way to make a long-term relationship work is to make it *work*. You don't expect unconditional love and acceptance and an amber-hued glow from your job, do you? From your city-league basketball team? From your ski weekends? (If you answer yes, turn immediately to the section entitled "Therapy-schmerapy" on page 41).

That's because anything of value in a man's life is going to be work. And that includes life with your sweetheart.

So pick up your socks, keep track of the remote control, throw out the video games that don't work but that contain a certain sentimental appeal because your fraternity brother "Bronto" threw up on them once. Do the dishes once in a while.

Is it that simple? No, but it will help a lot. So will listening, sharing, and trying to learn. To make getting along even easier, try to remember when you were starting out in your career and you were nothing but a bottom-feeding worm in the corporate food chain. (If you're still there, this exercise will be easier.) Think of your wife as a low-level colleague, a fellow worm. Think of the world as your oppressive, greedy, and unfeeling corporate overseer. You are united, shoulder to shoulder, worm belly to worm belly, heart to heart!

Now, when it comes time to choose sides, don't think of her as the woman who nags you to give up your Thursday-night backgammon game or as the person to whom you have pledged lifelong (farewell, Shanna!) fidelity. No, think of her as your fellow worm, squirming and battling with you as you take on the world. You are in this thing together.

Also, it's probably a good idea to have a vivid imagination when it comes to sex.

CHILDREN

Bundles of joy. Really expensive, demanding bundles of joy.

Not having children myself, I can nevertheless see the appeal of fatherhood, especially during those magical years when the little ones are old enough to fetch me food and drink, yet young enough to listen rapturously and wide-eyed about the time Daddy told the boss he hated the way workers were mistreated and underpaid, including him, and that's why Daddy doesn't go to the office anymore, and, "yes, little Billy, that's right, that's exactly why Daddy is just like Gandhi, except bigger and stronger. Now, how 'bout fetching me a beer, partner."

Of course, I can also see where a baby closely resembles a feeding machine with sloppy elimination habits who will suck net income for at least the next eighteen years while keeping mom too busy for sex.

Am I being unduly caustic about our world's future? Probably. Besides, based on the testimony of guy friends I trust, fatherhood is fun. These guys talk about "the moment my universe shifted on its axis." They mention "the most glorious kind of slavery." They say, "My child made me realize, for the first time, exactly who I was." They mention immortality, seeing the world through fresh eyes, the "exquisite pain" of watching their children grow up. Even though what the men have to say sounds an awful lot like the way I feel about psychedelic mushrooms, they seem sincere.

Refreshingly candid celebrity quote on
fatherhood that reveals an essential truth
about love, marriage, and infants
"It hasn't helped with the sex life. I get no time on the breasts anymore."

—John Tesh, musician, entertainer, television personality, and it must be pointed out, good father, referring half-jokingly to what the birth of his daughter, Prima, in 1994, meant to his marriage with actress Connie Sellecca

THE END

D·I·V·O·R·C·E.

Divorce is ugly, it's messy, and it's draining. Sometimes it's absolutely necessary. Other times, it represents weakness of moral fiber and the worst kind of narcissism. Why do you want one? (See "General Guidelines to Survive the Mystery and Madness of Love," page 129.)

Good luck.

BUYER'S GUIDE

LIVING LARGE
Barnes & Nobles
Stores across the country

Tower Records
Stores across the country

Barney Greengrass, the Sturgeon
    King
541 Amsterdam Ave.
New York, NY 10024
212-724-4707

Sherry Lehman Wine & Spirits
679 Madison Ave.
New York, NY
212-838-7500

LOOKING GOOD
Many of these stores have catalogs.
Call or write for details.

Turnbull & Asser*
71-72 Jermyn St.
London SW1, England
44-171-930-0502

Charvet*
28 Place Vendome
75001 Paris, France
33-1-42-60-30-70

Hilditch & Key*
73 Jermyn St.
London SW1, England
44-171-930-5336

*These three do fittings in the U.S.
Call or write for dates and cities.*

Ascot Chang
7 W. 57th St.
New York, NY 10019
1-800-486-9966
    and
9551-9553 Wilshire Blvd.
Los Angles, CA 90211
310-550-1309

David Lance, New York
42 E. 76th St.
New York, NY 10021
212-879-8686

Sulka
430 Park Ave.
New York, NY 10022
212-980-5226
*Branches in Chicago, San Francisco,
    Beverly Hills, Paris, and London*

Bergdorf Goodman
745 Fifth Ave.
New York, NY 10022
212-339-3255

New Republic
93 Spring St.
New York, NY 10012
212-219-3005

Worth & Worth
331 Madison Ave.
New York, NY 10017
212-867-6058

Bullock & Jones
340 Post St.
San Francisco, CA 94108
415-392-4243

Carroll & Company
425 North Canon Dr.
Beverly Hills, CA 90210
310-273-7974
1-800-238-9400 for catalog

Kiehl's
109 Third Ave.
New York, NY 10008
212-677-3171
1-800-KIEHLS1 for catalog

The Gap
They're everywhere.

FEELING STRONG
Paragon Sporting Goods
867 Broadway
New York, NY 10003
212-255-8036

Foot Locker
43 W. 34th St.
New York, NY 10001
212-971-9449
Stores across the country

Nike Town
669 North Michigan Ave.
Chicago, IL 60611
312-642-6363
    and
6 E. 57th St.
New York, NY 10022
212-891-6453

Whole Foods Market
2421 Broadway
New York, NY 10024
212-874-4000

Bally Total Fitness
1-800-846-0256
Locations across the country

LOVING WELL
Tiffany & Co
727 Fifth Ave.
New York, NY 10022
212-755-8000
1-800-526-0649 for catalog

Cartier Inc
2 E. 52nd St.
New York, NY 10022
212-753-0111
1-800-227-8437

1-800-Flowers
(1-800-356-9377)

Godiva Chocolatier Inc.
225 Liberty St.
New York, NY 10281
212-945-2174
1-800-9-GODIVA

Good Vibrations
1210 Valencia
San Francisco, CA 94110
415-974-8980
1-800-289-8423 for catalog

Victoria's Secret
34 E. 57th St.
New York, NY 10022
1-800-HER-GIFT for catalog
Stores across the country

INDEX